CONCUSSIONS

**Recent Titles in
Health and Medical Issues Today**

CONCUSSIONS

William Paul Meehan III

Health and Medical Issues Today

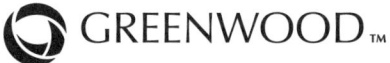

An Imprint of ABC-CLIO, LLC

Santa Barbara, California • Denver, Colorado

Library of Congress Cataloging-in-Publication Data

Names: Meehan, William Paul, author.
Title: Concussions / William Paul Meehan III.
Description: Santa Barbara, California : Greenwood, [2017] | Series: Health and medical issues today | Includes bibliographical references and index.
Identifiers: LCCN 2016033760 (print) | LCCN 2016036384 (ebook) | ISBN 9781440838941 (hardback) | ISBN 9781440838958 (ebook)
Subjects: LCSH: Brain—Concussion. | Brain—Concussion—Diagnosis. | Brain—Concussion—Prevention.
Classification: LCC RC394.C7 M374 2017 (print) | LCC RC394.C7 (ebook) | DDC 617.4/81044—dc23
LC record available at https://lccn.loc.gov/2016033760

ISBN: 978-1-4408-3894-1
EISBN: 978-1-4408-3895-8

21 20 19 18 17   2 3 4 5

This book is also available as an eBook.

Greenwood
An Imprint of ABC-CLIO, LLC

ABC-CLIO, LLC
130 Cremona Drive, P.O. Box 1911
Santa Barbara, California 93116-1911
www.abc-clio.com

This book is printed on acid-free paper ∞

Manufactured in the United States of America

for Marie, Billy, and Fionnuala

Contents

SERIES FOREWORD

Every day, the public is bombarded with information on developments in medicine and health care. Whether it is on the latest techniques in treatment or research, or on concerns over public health threats, this information directly affects the lives of people more than almost any other issue. Although there are many sources for understanding these topics—from websites and blogs to newspapers and magazines—students and ordinary citizens often need one resource that makes sense of the complex health and medical issues affecting their daily lives.

The *Health and Medical Issues Today* series provides just such a one-stop resource for obtaining a solid overview of the most controversial areas of health care in the 21st century. Each volume addresses one topic and provides a balanced summary of what is known. These volumes provide an excellent first step for students and lay people interested in understanding how health care works in our society today.

Each volume is broken into several sections to provide readers and researchers with easy access to the information they need:

Section I provides overview chapters on background information—including chapters on such areas as the historical, scientific, medical, social, and legal issues involved—that a citizen needs to intelligently understand the topic.

Section II provides capsule examinations of the most heated contemporary issues and debates, and analyzes in a balanced manner the viewpoints held by various advocates in the debates.

Section III provides a selection of reference material, such as annotated primary source documents, a timeline of important events, and

a directory of organizations that serve as the best next step in learning about the topic at hand.

The *Health and Medical Issues Today* series strives to provide readers
with all the information needed to begin making sense of some of the most
important debates going on in the world today. The series includes volumes on such topics as stem cell research, obesity, gene therapy, alternative medicine, organ transplantation, mental health, and more.

INTRODUCTION

Fans of the movies will recall scenes in which a boxer is given smelling salts as a means of reviving him and increasing his arousal after a concussion has left him dazed. While there is some poetic license exercised by the producers of such movies, it was not uncommon in past decades to see athletes revived after sustaining a concussion by smelling salts or other means, only to return to the same competition. Such a display would be highly criticized were it to occur nowadays.

Concussion, a form of traumatic brain injury, occurs commonly during sports, with studies suggesting that concussion accounts for approximately 13 percent of all injuries that occur during high school sports. Until recently, sport-related concussions were thought of as minor injuries of little consequence. In fact, official medical recommendations allowed for some athletes to return to competition 15 minutes after sustaining a concussion, so long as they reported their symptoms had resolved. Over the last two to three decades, however, attitudes about sport-related concussions have changed. Researchers have observed that some athletes seem to suffer symptoms from a concussion for days, weeks, even months. Moreover, brain function seems to diminish, temporarily, after a concussion for days, weeks, or even months. At times, brain function can be impaired even after athletes report their symptoms have resolved. In addition, concussions seem to have a cumulative effect, with repeated concussions resulting in more intense symptoms, worse brain function, and more pronounced signs of injury than first-time concussions.

Recently, some professional athletes, including American football players, ice hockey players, soccer players, and rugby players, among others, have started to speak out about the number of concussions they sustained during their careers and the symptoms they suffered as a result. Their openness has resulted in many stories about sport-related concussion in the public media. Nowadays, concussion is often in the news. In fact, it is hard to watch sporting events or follow the sports media for more than a few days without hearing the topic of concussion come up. This attention has led, gradually, to a recognition on the part of athletes, parents, coaches, physicians, and the American public in general that concussions should be treated more seriously. This increased awareness, however, has been accompanied by controversy and debate.

This book will define concussion, discuss the acute effects of concussion, describe the current treatment of concussions, outline the current concepts of the potential for long term and cumulative effects from concussion, and recount the research that has led to the modern understanding of concussions. Furthermore, this book will describe the current controversies surrounding concussions, sport-related concussions in particular. After completing this book, readers will be able to form their own knowledgeable, informed opinions about the controversies.

SECTION I

Overview

CHAPTER 1

Trauma-Induced Brain Dysfunction: Definition of Concussion

A logical place to begin a text on concussion is by defining concussion, describing what exactly a concussion is. Defining concussion, however, is harder than you might think. Concussion has been defined differently by different medical organizations and medical societies over the last 30 years. These varying definitions have made it difficult for researchers to compare studies and for doctors to determine the best treatments for patients. In an effort to standardize the definition, an international consensus on concussion in sports has been assembled and has met several times, most recently in Zürich, Switzerland, in November 2012. At that conference, experts defined concussion as follows:

> Concussion is a brain injury and is defined as a complex pathophysiological process affecting the brain, induced by biomechanical forces. Several common features that incorporate clinical, pathologic and biomechanical injury constructs that may be utilized [sic] in defining the nature of a concussive head injury include:
>
> 1. Concussion may be caused either by a direct blow to the head, face, neck or elsewhere on the body with an "impulsive" force transmitted to the head.
> 2. Concussion typically results in the rapid onset of short-lived impairment of neurological function that resolves spontaneously. However, in some cases, symptoms and signs may evolve over a number of minutes to hours.

3. Concussion may result in neuropathological changes, but the acute clinical symptoms largely reflect a functional disturbance rather than a structural injury and, as such, no abnormality is seen on standard structural neuroimaging studies.
4. Concussion results in a graded set of clinical symptoms that may or may not involve loss of consciousness. Resolution of the clinical and cognitive symptoms typically follows a sequential course. However, it is important to note that in some cases symptoms may be prolonged (Consensus Statement on Concussion in Sport: The 4th International Conference on Concussion in Sport, Zurich, *J Athl Train.* 2013 Jul–Aug; 48(4):554–75).

Although this definition may be useful for researchers, scientists, physicians, and other clinicians, it is full of medical jargon and, therefore, does not result in a true understanding of concussion for most people. Perhaps a simpler way to define concussion is "trauma-induced brain dysfunction." That is to say, a concussion is when the brain temporarily stops functioning properly as a result of trauma. This temporary dysfunction of the brain results in the symptoms associated with concussion. Symptoms are the problems and abnormal feelings experienced by a person who has suffered a concussion. Some of the more typical symptoms of concussion are headaches, dizziness, nausea, confusion, amnesia, sensitivity to light, sensitivity to noise, difficulty with concentration, difficulty with memory, and the overall feelings of being slowed down (Table 1.1).

Table 1.1 Symptoms of Concussion

- Headache
- Dizziness/unsteadiness
- Difficulty concentrating
- Vision changes/sensitivity to light
- Nausea or vomiting
- Drowsiness
- Amnesia
- Sensitivity to noise
- Ringing in the ears
- Irritability
- Feeling "out of it"
- Trouble falling asleep
- Sleeping more than usual
- Difficulty remembering
- Feeling slowed down
- Increased emotionality
- Feeling as if "in a fog"

The symptoms of concussion should be distinguished from the signs associated with concussion. Signs are findings that can be perceived by others when observing a person who has sustained a concussion. Some of the typical signs of concussion are poor balance, loss of consciousness, confusion, repetitive questioning (whereby the person with a concussion repeatedly asks the same question over and over again, despite being given the answer), and acting confused, among others (Table 1.2).

Loss of consciousness deserves special attention. Historically, physicians and scientists were uncertain as to whether or not blows to the head that resulted in a loss of consciousness caused the same injury as blows to the head that resulted in imbalance, headaches, confusion, and other symptoms but did not result in a loss of consciousness. This led to the use of different terms for these injuries, with some people using the term "concussion" only when a loss of consciousness occurred. We now know that, while a loss of consciousness can be a very dramatic sign of concussion, it is relatively uncommon and occurs with only 5 to 10 percent of concussions that occur during sports. Thus, most sport-related concussions occur without a loss of consciousness.

In addition to producing signs and symptoms, concussion also results in problems of cognition. The word *cognition* refers to the activities of the mind, such as thinking, learning, remembering, and understanding. After a concussion, cognition is adversely affected such that the acts of thinking, understanding, learning, and remembering are more difficult. This can be observed when speaking with those who have sustained concussions, as they may be slow to think, slow to respond, and unable to recall simple facts such as where they are, what day of the week it is, what year it is, what the score of the game in which they are playing is, or who the team they are playing against is.

Table 1.2 Signs of Concussion

- Walking off-balance
- Appearing dazed
- Acting confused
- Inability to recall score of current game
- Unable to recall opponent
- Forgetting game rules or play assignments
- Slow verbal responses
- Increased or inappropriate emotionality
- Poor physical coordination
- Acting disoriented

Concussion directly affects balance and coordination. When athletes sustain concussions, this poor balance and coordination may be noticed by teammates, coaches, referees, and spectators, as athletes may be slow to rise, appear unsteady, or even fall over. They may fumble with objects they are trying to manipulate. They may have difficulty performing the duties required for their sport.

Importantly, our definition of concussion, "trauma-induced brain dysfunction," emphasizes the fact that concussion is largely a functional problem. Most readers will think of an injury as resulting in structural damage to body tissues, such as bruises, cuts, scrapes, or lacerations. Concussion, however, is not so much a structural injury, represented by damage to tissues, as a functional disturbance. When the brain of a person who has sustained a concussion is examined by using modern-day imaging techniques, such as computed tomography (CT) or magnetic resonance imaging (MRI), to obtain pictures of the brain, the brain appears uninjured. In fact, it appears perfectly normal; there is no bruising, no bleeding, no cells dying. Although structurally normal in appearance, the brain that has sustained a concussion is not functioning properly: reaction times are slower, memory is poorer, and the ability to concentrate is diminished. Thus, when diagnosing a patient with a concussion, doctors rely heavily on the symptoms of concussion reported by the patient and assessments of brain function, as opposed to pictures of the brain. The next chapter explains why the brain is not functioning properly after a concussion, despite the lack of gross structural injury.

SUMMARY

Concussion, a form of traumatic brain injury, is a temporary state of brain dysfunction caused by trauma that results in symptoms such as headache, dizziness, or nausea, and signs such as imbalance, slowed speech, loss of consciousness, or repetitive questioning. A concussion is not a typical structural injury, such as a bruise or scrape, but rather a disturbance of brain function that results in slower reaction times, poorer memory, and poor balance, among other difficulties.

CHAPTER 2

Biomechanics and Pathophysiology

Explaining how concussions occur and how they affect the brain may result in greater understanding than simply trying to define concussion. In order to explain a concussion, however, we first have to learn about the basic anatomy of the brain—how it is shaped and where it is in the body. Furthermore, we need a basic understanding of how the brain works normally, its physiology.

First, let us review the basic anatomy of the brain. The brain is a complex structure that, although shaped differently, is approximately the size of an average grapefruit. The human brain weighs approximately 3 pounds and is approximately 15 cm in length, along its longest axis. It consists mostly of water and fat, giving it a soft, malleable consistency similar to tofu. The brain has multiple folds, or sulci, that give its surface a convoluted appearance. It is housed inside the skull, just above the roof of the mouth. The skull, which is made of thick, hard bone, protects the brain from direct impact or trauma.

On a microscopic level, the brain consists of cells. In particular, the brain is the home of billions of nerve cells, or neurons, which are essential to brain function. Neurons consist of four main parts: the dendrites, the cell body, the axon, and the terminal end. They vary in length from very short, less than 1 mm, to very long, longer than 1 m. Some neurons travel from the brain down the back in what is known as the spinal cord. There are also neurons that course from the spinal cord to the muscles and other organs of the body, regulating muscle movement and other bodily functions.

Now, let us review the physiology or the neurons, the way they normally function. The neurons of an uninjured, normally functioning brain work by sending signals to one another. This signaling is accomplished by neurons conducting an action potential. An action potential can be difficult to understand the first time you learn about it. I like to use an example from everyday life to illustrate the basic principal. Most readers are familiar with the movement of a rope when one end is lifted up and then rapidly accelerated downward. A hump forms at the end of the rope closest to the person handling it, and then rapidly travels down to the opposite end of the rope. In effect, the impulse started by the person moving the rope has travelled down the length of the rope to the opposite end. An action potential works similarly, by transmitting a signal from one end of the neuron, the cell body, down the length of the axon, to the opposite end. But instead of the rope moving up and down, an action potential involves sodium ions moving in and out of the cell membrane very rapidly all the way down to the other end of the neuron.

In its normal, resting state, when the neuron is not performing any specific function, there are molecules of sodium and potassium surrounding its membrane. Specifically, sodium molecules are highly concentrated outside of the cell, while potassium molecules are highly concentrated inside the cell. When a neuron conducts an action potential, channels in the membrane open, allowing sodium to move from the outside of the cell through the open channel and into the cell. These channels are known as the sodium-potassium channels. During an action potential, the sodium-potassium channels closest to the cell body open first, followed by the channels a little further down the axon, followed by the channels still further down the axon, and so on, all the way down the length of the axon until the sodium-potassium channels at the far end open, allowing sodium to rush into the terminal end. When sodium rushes into the terminal end, it causes the neuron to release a chemical. When the chemical is detected by the adjacent neuron, the adjacent neuron conducts an action potential of its own.

As I said, an action potential can be difficult to understand the first time you learn about it. Spend some time rereading the last two paragraphs a few times until you get it. It is essential to understand this aspect of how neurons work, in order to understand what happens at the time of a concussion.

BIOMECHANICS OF CONCUSSION

Concussion is caused by an acceleration of the brain. Acceleration is really the process of moving faster, increasing in speed, or changing direction. Typically, concussion occurs after the head is struck, causing it to accelerate away from the direction of whatever struck it.

While we now know that acceleration is what results in concussion, it was not always that clear.

Researchers during the 1940s were conducting experiments in animals to try and determine what caused concussion. In order to cause a concussion, they struck the animals in the head with a weight that was attached to a pendulum. These researchers noticed that if the head was held still at the time it was struck, it would not cause a concussion as often as when the head was allowed to move freely, or accelerate, after being struck. Thus, these researchers determined it was the acceleration itself—the moving of the brain from a state of motionless rest to acceleration—that caused the concussion.

There are, however, two main types of acceleration: linear and rotational. Linear acceleration is when an object moves from a state of motionless rest to a state of motion in a straight, linear direction. A common example of this can be seen on the roads. A car stopped at a red light is in a state of motionless rest. When the light turns green, the car accelerates in a straight line through the intersection. Rotational acceleration is when an object moves from a state of motionless rest to a state of rotational motion or spinning. A common example of this can be seen when children play with a toy top. When the top is resting on the floor, it is in a state of motionless rest. When a child grabs the stem between the thumb and forefinger and gives it a spin, the toy top rotationally accelerates, spinning around and around. Once scientists realized that concussions resulted from acceleration, they began conducting further experiments to determine which type of acceleration, linear or rotational, was more likely to cause a concussion.

In a widely cited medical paper, a physicist named Holbourn considered the physical properties of the brain, noting that the brain consists mostly of water. Therefore, he hypothesized that the brain might act similarly to water. He pointed out that, if one were to fill a clear flask half with water, and place some shredded cotton on top of the water in order to more easily see how the water moves, and then push the flask in a straight line, there would be minimal disruption of the water and cotton pieces. The cotton, water, and flask would all move together, as one object. If, however, the flask was spun or rotated, the flask would move, but the bulk of the water would stay still. At a closer level, the molecules of water adjacent to the flask would be pulled along with the spinning flask, while the molecules of water closer to the center would remain motionless. There would be a shear strain applied to the adjacent water molecules, a shearing between the molecules of water next to the glass and those closer to the center. Holbourn argued that if the brain is made mostly of water and its physical properties are therefore similar to water, the brain, when rotated, should experience a similar shear strain. He made an analogy between the flask full of water and a skull containing a brain. If the skull were subjected to a linear acceleration, the brain would be minimally affected. But, if the skull were subjected to a rotational acceleration, the brain would be subjected to a shear strain that could result in injury. Thus, he proposed that rotational acceleration was more likely to cause a concussion than linear acceleration. Still, debate continued.

While recognizing the value of the analogy, some scientists pointed out the brain, while similar in its physical properties to water, was a highly complex structure that could not be reduced to a simple model. Therefore, more experiments needed to be conducted. Furthermore, most of the time, when the head is struck, it accelerates in both a linear and rotational manner. When a boxer is struck on the chin, his head both accelerates linearly in the direction opposite the blow, and also spins or rotates away from the blow. It is difficult to separate purely linear from purely rotational acceleration. In a key experiment published in the 1970s, two scientists, Ayub K. Ommaya and T.A. Gennarelli, did just that. They divided monkeys into two groups of 12. All monkeys were placed in a helmet that was attached to a piston operated by a motor. When the machine was activated, it would accelerate the head of a monkey over the distance of 1 inch. For 12 of the monkeys, the head was accelerated in a straight line over the distance of 1 inch. For the other 12 monkeys, the head was rotated over an arc of 1 inch. In both groups, the same amount of force was used to accelerate the head. In this way, they were able to isolate the effects due to rotational acceleration from those due to linear acceleration. Their results were telling.

All the monkeys that experienced purely rotational acceleration were immediately knocked unconscious. None of the monkeys that experienced purely linear acceleration was knocked unconscious. The experiments showed definitively that rotational acceleration contributes more to concussion than linear. Furthermore, there was no blow or trauma to the head of the monkeys in Ommaya and Gennarelli's experiments, underscoring the fact that it is not the blow or trauma itself that produces a concussion, but the rotational acceleration of the head after the blow.

As noted above, in most circumstances outside the controlled setting of a laboratory, when a force is transmitted to the head, both types of acceleration occur—linear and rotational. But given the findings of Ommaya and Gennarelli, it seems the rotational acceleration is what results in a concussion. This can be observed in sports, particularly in combat sports such as mixed martial arts. Often, in mixed martial arts, concussion is caused by a blow to the chin. Remember that the brain sits at the top of the skull, above the cheekbones. Therefore, a blow to the chin does not have any direct impact on the brain itself. It does, however, result in a fairly rapid spinning or rotational acceleration of the brain. This spinning is what results in the concussion.

While most commonly concussion occurs after a direct blow to the head, particularly in sports, direct trauma to the head is not necessary to cause a concussion. One can imagine that a blow delivered somewhere else on the body may result in a rapid spinning of the brain and therefore result in a concussion despite the fact that the head itself is not struck. A classic example of this would be a passenger riding in a car while wearing a seatbelt around both the lap and shoulder. If the car strikes a stationary object and stops suddenly, momentum carries the passenger forward. Since the body is restrained by the shoulder and lap belt, it will move relatively little. The head, which is unrestrained, however, will continue to move forward and will spin with the chin moving down towards the chest. This type of rotational acceleration may result in a concussion, despite the fact that the head itself was not struck.

While it is helpful to know that rotational acceleration results in concussion, we have not yet discussed why—why would spinning of the brain result in any dysfunction at all? In order to understand why, we first need to understand how the brain normally works. Recall from earlier in this chapter that the brain consists of millions of brain cells called neurons. Each neuron consists for four main parts: the dendrites, the cell body, the axon, and the terminal end. Neurons work by transmitting signals to one another and to other cells of the body. These signals are facilitated by something called an action potential. During an action potential, a signal is transmitted from the cell body, down the length of the axon, to the terminal end. Once this signal reaches the terminal end, the neuron releases a chemical that causes the neurons next to it to fire their own action potential. Also, recall that action potentials rely on the movement of sodium ions, which are usually located outside the cell, through channels in the cell membrane into the axon.

To illustrate the whole process, let us use an example. Say I decide to kick a soccer ball. Somehow, a message must be conducted from my mind, which has decided to kick the ball, to my leg muscles, which will do the actual kicking of the ball. That message is sent from neurons to muscles cells through a series of action potentials. Before I decide to kick the ball, the neurons are in their resting state. In a normal resting state, the fluid around the neurons contains sodium ions. These sodium ions do not move into the cell because they cannot get through the cell membrane. When I decide to kick a ball, however, channels in the cell membrane nearest to the cell body open, allowing sodium to move into the cell. As these ions move into the cell, they trigger the opening of channels downstream from them along the axon to open. When those holes open, they trigger holes downstream from them to open. This continues, very rapidly, down the entire length of the axon and into the terminal end. When holes in the cell membrane of the terminal end open, sodium flows into the terminal end triggering the release of a chemical. The released chemical is then taken up by the next neuron, triggering its own signal or action potential. This signal is transmitted from neuron to neuron by a series of action potentials, all the way down the spinal cord, out through the nerves, and eventually to the leg muscles, causing the muscles to contract and kick the soccer ball.

THAT IS HOW THE BRAIN USUALLY WORKS

Rapid spinning of the brain causes the brain, temporarily, to stop working properly by interfering with the ability of the cells to fire action potentials. This temporary dysfunction is what we call a concussion. Here is how it happens. When the brain is spun rapidly, not all parts of the brain are moving at the same speed. Thus, the brain undergoes a shear strain, as previously described by Holbourn, causing the brain to deform. Much like when a bowl of Jello is spun rapidly, it deforms and starts to jiggle, when the brain is spun rapidly, it is deformed by the acceleration. This deformation causes channels within the cell membranes of neurons to deform also. When they are deformed, they open, allowing massive amounts of sodium to rush into the cells. As sodium rushes in, an action potential is initiated. This process is indiscriminant, meaning it is not just the cells that are meant to fire action potentials, but any cell exposed to the shear strain caused by the rotational acceleration of the brain will fire an action potential. Furthermore, during a normal action potential, only a small amount of sodium moves across the cell membrane, but when a concussion occurs, a relatively massive amount of sodium rushes into the cell. Sodium gets stuck inside of the cell and the cell cannot function properly, or fire another action potential, until all that sodium is pumped back out.

Sodium is pumped back out by a protein in the cell membrane known as the sodium-potassium pump. Since the main function of the sodium-potassium pump is to pump sodium out after an action potential, which usually involves relatively small amounts of sodium, the pumps are overwhelmed by the massive amount of sodium that rushes in during a concussion. The sodium-potassium pump is powered by the common energy molecules adenosine triphosphate, more commonly known as ATP.

ATP is the energy molecule of the body. It supplies the energy that allows brain cells to think, the heart to pump, the lungs to breathe, muscle cells to contract, and really all the cells of the body to function. ATP is ultimately derived from the food we eat and is delivered to the cells of the brain through the bloodstream. Unfortunately, for a period of a day to weeks after a concussion, there is decreased blood flow to the brain. Therefore, after a concussion occurs, the brain needs more ATP in order to pump sodium out of the brain cells so that they can function properly, but less ATP is being delivered because there is less blood flow to the brain. This mismatch of supply and demand results in the prolongation of concussion symptoms.

It should be noted that while this is one of the more commonly accepted hypotheses regarding concussion, there are other hypotheses to explain what takes place for concussion. But for the sake of simplicity, we will not discuss the other hypotheses.

SUMMARY

Concussion results from a rapid spinning or rotational acceleration of the brain. When the brain spins, a shear strain can deform the neurons, allowing large amounts of sodium ions to move into the cells, which then fire action potentials indiscriminately. Until these cells pump sodium back out, they cannot function properly. This dysfunction results in the signs and symptoms of concussion. Thus, concussion is largely a problem of brain function, as opposed to a gross structural injury. The brain requires ATP in order to heal, but there is less ATP being delivered to the brain, as there is decreased blood flow to the brain.

CHAPTER 3

History of Sport-Related Concussion

As far back as 600 years before Christ, people have engaged in sports and athletic competitions that carried with them an increased risk of concussion. Sports such as wrestling and fist fighting were common and were commonly viewed by spectators even at the Olympics. The symptoms of concussion were described by Hippocrates himself, the ancient Greek physician who is often described as the father of medicine. Writings from Hippocrates note that "In cerebral concussion, whatever the cause, the patient becomes speechless, . . . falls down immediately, loses their [sic] speech, cannot see and hear" (Zillmer, Shneider, Tinker, and Kaminaris 2006).

Other well-known physicians of long-ago times have also commented on and described concussions that occurred during sports. In the first century AD, an Arabic physician, Rhazes, described concussion as a problem of brain function in the absence of gross structural injury. It is often simpler for people to think of injuries as damage to the actual tissues of the body. As described earlier, however, concussion is largely a disturbance of brain function as opposed to damage to the structure of the brain itself. As Rhazes described this distinction in the first century AD, it is perhaps surprising that this distinction is still not understood by many people today who consider sport-related concussion a bruise of the brain.

During the Middle Ages, physicians noted that, in general, athletes who sustain concussions in sports seem to recover quite quickly and without any long-term problems. They noted the distinction between these good outcomes for athletes who sustained a concussion during sports, compared to those who sustained direct injury to the cells of the brain. During the Middle Ages, sports such as jousting were quite common. Jousting can result in skull fracture and direct penetration of the brain by the lance. When this occurred, physicians noted that athletes were more likely to have long-term problems as a result of these brain injuries when compared to athletes who sustained a concussion.

They also noted at this time that problems with speech and memory were common after a sport-related concussion, in addition to the more obvious symptoms of dizziness, imbalance, and frank loss of consciousness.

During the 18th and 19th centuries, physicians began to further their understanding of concussion by attempting to describe what was taking place at the cellular level, what was occurring in the brain cells that led to the observed dysfunction, signs, and symptoms experienced by the athlete. They began to develop hypotheses about the cellular causes of the signs and symptoms of concussion. Many of the hypotheses developed during the 18th and 19th centuries contributed to the hypothesis discussed in the earlier chapter that is currently one of the most common understandings of concussion today.

It is around this same time that physicians began to question the causes of the symptoms of concussion. Since it had become more firmly established that athletes experiencing symptoms of concussion had no gross structural injuries or abnormalities to the brain tissue itself, physicians and others began to speculate that perhaps the symptoms were the result of a feigning or faking by people who wanted to avoid work or other duties, or who were perhaps motivated by a lawsuit, in an attempt to collect some financial benefit over an incidence that had occurred.

In the early 1900s, American football had evolved into a game that many considered violent and aggressive. There was great debate and controversy regarding the aggression and physical, even brutal, nature of sports. Young men were being killed while playing American football, including young men from some of the finest universities. This problem captured the attention of the leaders of these universities and even government officials of the day, up to and including the president of the United States of America. In an effort to decrease the number of young men being killed while participating in football and, in part, to attempt to save the game from all the negative publicity, President Theodore Roosevelt called a conference of leaders at these institutions to a meeting. This group formed the Intercollegiate Athletic Association, which ultimately devolved into the modern-day National Collegiate Athletic Association. Through changes to the rules, equipment, and other adaptations, the game was made safer in the sense that fewer young men were dying as a result of participation.

Also in the 1900s, physicians started to describe a clinical condition in boxers. Some boxers, most often boxers who were known for their ability to "take a punch" and as a result absorb multiple blows to their heads over the course of their careers, were noted to have changes later in life that included unsteady gait, slowed muscular responses, mental confusion, difficulties with speech, physical tremors particularly of the fingers, dragging of the leg and foot while walking, and even facial characteristics described as "masked-like facies," where there was decreased expression notable in the face similar to what is currently seen in other diseases such as Parkinson's disease. One of the early describers of this condition, Dr. Harrison Martland, noted that it seemed to be more common in fighters who were not particularly successful and were used mostly for training purposes. These boxers, therefore, had a long exposure to blows of the head. The collection of symptoms observed in these former boxers became known as punch-drunk syndrome or, at other times, dementia pugilistic. Other terms have been used to describe this condition, up to and including the more modern-day term chronic traumatic encephalopathy (CTE).

As the 19th century progressed, physicians began to study the brains of these boxers and noted that they appeared different than the brains of individuals who were not suffering these symptoms and who were not exposed to repeated trauma to the head.

In 1984, Saunders and Harbaugh described the case of a 19-year-old college football player who sustained a concussion during a fistfight. He had headaches and nausea following his injury, such that he spent some time in the college infirmary. Several days after his injury, he felt better, but still complained of a mild headache. He returned to football and, despite not sustaining any unusual head trauma, he collapsed, losing consciousness. He was taken to a local hospital where he underwent heroic measures in an attempt to save his life. Despite these efforts, he ultimately died; at his autopsy, he was noted to have massive swelling of his brain. The brain swelled so much that it filled the entirety of his skull and started to get forced out the hole in the bottom of his skull, which normally allows for the spinal cord to descend into the neck, due to the pressure. As it was forced through this hole, the brain was crushed, rendering the nerves ineffective. He was unable to breathe on his own and succumbed to the injury. As you would expect, this case raised awareness within the medical community about the potential effects of returning to sports, particularly American football, prior to full recovery from concussion. The case raised the concern that, perhaps, the brain is more susceptible to trauma, even minor trauma, when it is incompletely recovered from a prior injury. The suffering of brain swelling and death from minor trauma sustained while still recovering from a previous injury has been termed "second impact syndrome."

Well into the second half of the 20th century, neuropsychologists began to study the effects of concussion on memory, the speed with which athletes process their thoughts, reaction time, and symptoms experienced by the athlete. They made several key discoveries. They noted that concussion caused problems with cognition that lasted beyond the first few minutes to hours, lasting longer than was previously thought. They also noted that, at times, athletes' symptoms would resolve, yet their cognitive dysfunction would continue. Around the same time, other investigators noted that balance was affected by concussion and imbalance lasted more than the first few minutes or days. Studies revealed that athletes who had experienced concussions in the past were more likely to experience sport-related concussions in the future than their teammates or opponents who had not previously experienced a concussion. Furthermore, athletes who had prior sport-related concussions seemed to have cumulative effects. Athletes who sustained previous concussions were more likely to lose consciousness with future injuries than athletes who had not sustained prior concussions. Athletes with prior concussions were more likely to suffer amnesia, have a longer duration of symptoms, and have a greater intensity of symptoms with their future concussions than athletes who had no previous concussion.

Toward the end of the 20th century, the findings and abnormalities of the brains of boxers who had dementia pugilistica were noted among former American football players. Many of these players had experienced difficulty with memory, including dementia, as well as mood swings, headaches, and multiple other problems later in life. Hypotheses were developed about the connection between the trauma to the head sustained during American football, the findings of the brains noted at autopsy, and the problems the athletes were experiencing later in life. This ultimately led to several high-profile athletes retiring from American football due to concerns over the concussions they had sustained and the problems that had been observed in older athletes later in life.

All of these findings resulted in a substantial amount of public attention and started changing the way Americans thought about sport-related concussion. Prior to the late 20th century and early 21st century, most people viewed sport-related concussions as inconsequential. It was believed that athletes had some brief signs or symptoms that resolved completely and fully, and most athletes were returned to sport within a few days, even the same day on many occasions. But, given the findings described above, views began to change. People became more concerned about sport-related concussions and about the potential for longer-term effects or even permanent effects. This led to considerable debate and controversy, as often occurs when a way of thinking begins to change. Many people still feel that concussions are short-lived and inconsequential without residual effects. Indeed, this was the thinking for centuries and some recent evidence, they argue, should not change our thinking. Others are more concerned and believe that concussions can have effects that last for days, weeks, even months, and, perhaps, can be permanent.

Driven in part by the concern over long-term effects from sport-related concussions including traumatic encephalopathy, there were calls to ban collision sports such as American football and combat sports such as boxing and mixed martial arts, forbidding their participation. Others have called simply for banning participation by children in these sports. Still others argue that, even if the risks are legitimate, they are relatively low, noting that most people who participate in contact and collision sports do not go on to develop CTE. Many people argue that a bigger problem facing American children today is inactivity, which leads to an increased risk of heart disease, increased risk of stroke, and many other health problems. The risks of these health problems can be reduced by participation in athletics, including American football, and therefore sports should not be banned.

Furthermore, there is still debate regarding the long-term effects of having sustained multiple concussions in sports. Many people believe that the concussions sustained during sports are leading to depression, headaches, mood or behavior problems, difficulties with memory, dementia, and other symptoms that not only last, but also in many cases do not appear until later in life. Others believe that many middle-aged and older men who never participated in contact or collision sports develop depression, mood and behavior problems, troubles with their memory, and some progress to frank dementia. Therefore, we should not automatically attribute those signs and symptoms to participation in sports. All this debate has led to changes in the way athletes who sustain concussions are managed. This has led to laws in all the 50 states in the United States regarding the management of athletes who sustain concussions. It has led to changes in the rules of the games and in the medical protocols used for treating athletes. Indeed, many high school readers of this text will be surprised to hear that concussion was recently considered a trivial injury without long-term consequences. Those readers who have parents 40 years of age or older, however, will readily learn from their parents that there was a lack of concern over sport-related concussions during their childhood and early adulthood. They now see a dramatic difference in the way concussion is viewed by Americans.

SUMMARY

Sport-related concussion has been a well-known entity since the time of Hippocrates. Much has been learned by the observations of physicians throughout time. Discoveries made through medicine and science have led to a change in the way concussion is viewed by athletes and the public at large. Concerns have led to changes in the way games are played, the way athletes are managed, and even laws and public policies designed to protect athletes from any potential consequences of injuries sustained during sports. As often happens, however, these discoveries have led to much debate and controversy as the evidence is limited in what it tells us and interpretations vary.

CHAPTER 4

The Epidemiology of Concussion

Concussion has been identified as a major health problem in the United States and globally by such organizations as the Centers for Disease Control and Prevention (CDC) in the United States and the World Health Organization. Worldwide, an estimated 42 million people sustain concussions annually. Studies estimate that approximately 2 million medical visits each year in the United States are for concussions. And since many people who sustain a concussion do not report to their doctor's office or the emergency room, there are many more occurring that have not been included in large studies. In fact, the CDC estimates that as many as 3.8 million traumatic brain injuries may occur each year in sports alone, most of them being concussion.

Concussions occur most commonly as a result of motor vehicle collisions, falls, sports participation, and assault. The incidence of concussion varies based on age, gender, geography, and other factors. For example, concussions sustained by young children and the elderly more commonly result from falls, whereas older children, adolescents, and younger adults more commonly sustain concussions during motor vehicles collisions or sports participation.

Sport-related concussions are unique in several ways. First, since athletes represent an organized, readily identifiable group who are at known risk of sustaining concussions, they are often the subjects of medical research. Thus, much of what we have learned about concussion we owe to the athletes who have been willing to participate in these studies. Second, the forces involved in sport-related concussion tend to be lower than those involved in motor vehicles, assaults, and falls, particularly falls from a height. Third, participation in sports is optional. Most of us have no choice but to leave the house to attend school or go to work. For many, this requires transportation on a bicycle, in a car, on a bus, or by subway. But athletes choose to play sports. They could easily spend their time, instead, playing music or reading books. Furthermore, athletes choose which sports they play. Since the incidence of injures varies by sports, athletes could use the data regarding the incidence of concussion in different sports to help make decisions about which sports they wish to participate in. Finally, studies of concussions that occur during sports can tell us when during a given sporting event concussions are most likely to occur and which types of situations are more likely to result in concussions. This data could then be used to develop ways of preventing concussions. Therefore, we will discuss the occurrence of concussions in several common sports.

COMBAT SPORTS

Combat sports are those sports in which opponents are in a controlled, organized, fight with each other. Sports such as boxing, wrestling, karate, and mixed martial arts are typical combat sports. Boxing and mixed martial arts are distinct from wrestling, as blows to the head are an accepted and even encouraged part of the sport. Indeed, one of the main goals of the sports is to give the opponent a concussion, which may rapidly lead to the winning of the bout. The numerous blows to the head delivered during these sports, the nonspecific nature of concussion symptoms, the desire to appear tough to one's opponents, and the variation between boxers in their ability to "take a punch" (absorb a punch to the face without developing visible signs of concussion) makes determining the actual incidence of concussion in boxing and mixed martial arts difficult. It is safe to say, however, that concussions occur commonly in combat sports, particularly those that encourage blows to the head, with some studies suggesting that in 1 out of every 10 bouts, a mixed martial arts fighter experiences a concussion.

AMERICAN FOOTBALL

While the occurrence of concussions in sports is becoming widely recognized, American football clearly garners most of the attention, perhaps due to the hard-hitting, fast-moving nature of the game or perhaps due to its popularity. Each year, there are nearly 2 million participants in American football, with 1.5 million in high school. Studies of high school and college athletes suggest that American football has one of the highest incidence rates of concussion in sports. These studies, however, may vastly underestimate the incidence of concussion in American football because they rely on athletes reporting their injuries. Several studies have shown that only about half of American football players who sustain concussions report their injuries. The rest continue to play, without alerting anyone.

ICE HOCKEY

Although less attention is paid to the concussions that occur in ice hockey when compared to those that occur during American football, several studies suggest that the incidence of concussions in ice hockey is comparable to that of American football, with some studies suggesting a higher incidence in ice hockey. Although male ice hockey is a collision sport, a sport during which routine, purposeful, body-to-body collisions occur as a legal and expected part of the game, and female ice hockey is a contact (but not collision) sport, a sport during which body-to-body contact occurs as a recognized part of the game, but purposeful body-to-body collisions are not allowed, some studies have suggested the incidence of concussion is comparable between the two and may be even higher in female ice hockey.

LACROSSE

Like American football and male ice hockey, male lacrosse is a collision sport. Male lacrosse carries the third highest incidence of concussion (after American football and male ice hockey) among high school team sports. Although female lacrosse is a contact but noncollision sport, some studies suggest the incidence of concussion is comparable to that of male lacrosse.

RUGBY

Rugby is unique in that it is a collision sport for which the rules are nearly the same for both male and female athletes. Concussions in rugby not only occur most often with body-to-body collisions during the act of tackling, but they also occur when the athlete's head strikes the ground. Concussions are common during illegal play, with some studies suggesting concussion accounts for 40 percent of all injuries that occur during illegal play.

SOCCER

Although considered a generally safe sport, the incidence of concussion in soccer, particularly female soccer, is quite high. In fact, for female team sports, soccer carries one of the highest incidences of concussion. Soccer is unique, as the head is used to strike the ball and propel it down the field. This use of the head often results in the head being placed in a vulnerable position where it may be struck by the head or body of an opponent, the fist of a goalkeeper, or the goalposts. Furthermore, when collisions occur in the air, players can be knocked off balance and fall striking their head on the playing surface. In addition, falls that occur when legs become tangled or a player is slide tackled can also result in concussions.

BASKETBALL

The rules of basketball are similar for male and female players. Concussions during basketball occur when contact is made with another player or after a fall on the court. The incidence of concussion seems to be similar for male and female players, although some studies suggest a higher incidence for female athletes.

BASEBALL/SOFTBALL

Baseball and softball are safe sports, including with regards to concussions, as the incidence is relatively low. Still, concussions occur in each when a player is struck with the ball, collides with another player, or collides with a stationary object such as the outfield wall.

SKIING AND SNOWBOARDING

Downhill or alpine snow sports involve large numbers of amateur athletes travelling at high rates of speed surrounded by other snow sports enthusiasts and stationary obstacles such as trees, chair lift poles, moguls, and ice patches. Despite the risk involved, concussions are relatively uncommon when compared to some of the other sports we have discussed. Still, they occur, often when a skier or snowboarder collides with another person on the slopes or with a stationary object.

CHEERLEADING

Over the last several decades, cheerleading has changed from a relatively safe activity during which cheerleaders literally led the cheers of the crowd, to a vigorous sport that combines the skills of acrobatics, gymnastics, weightlifting, and dancing. Modern cheerleaders often perform aerial stunts, 20 feet in the air, without the safety of netting or pads to land on.

Along with the transformation, the incidence of concussion has increased dramatically. Furthermore, cheerleading is unique as a sport during which the incidence of concussion is higher during practice than competition. This likely reflects the nature of these two activities. Practice is when cheerleaders are learning and practicing new stunts, which they have yet to perfect. Performance tends to involve stunts that cheerleaders are confident they can perform well without making a mistake.

Summary

Concussions occur in nearly all sports, and are the most common neurological injury in sports, although the frequency with which they occur varies between different sports. As might be expected, collision sports, during which routine, purposeful, body-to-body collisions occur as a legal and expected part of the game, carry the highest risk of concussion. Among sports that have similar rules for male and female athletes, studies suggest females may have a higher risk of sustaining concussions.

CHAPTER 5

Diagnosis and Assessment

Since the brain with a concussion cannot fire action potentials and, therefore, cannot work properly, patients who have concussions have temporary difficulties using their brains effectively. Their reaction time is slowed; they take longer to think and process information; they have poorer memories than usual; they have poorer balance than usual; and they experience other common signs and symptoms of concussion. When doctors are evaluating patients who may have suffered concussions, they assess several domains, including symptoms, balance, and cognitive difficulties.

As explained earlier, symptoms are those abnormal feelings experienced by the patient who has a concussion; signs are those abnormalities that can be seen and evaluated by others when looking at a person with a concussion. In order to help assess the symptoms experienced by the patient suffering from a concussion, several groups and organizations have developed symptom scales or symptom inventories that allow patients to report which symptoms they have while rating the degree to which they are experiencing each symptom. One of the more common symptom scales was developed by the international consensus on concussion in sports and is part of the overall Sport Concussion Assessment Tool, which is now on its third version (SCAT 3). The SCAT symptom scale lists a total of 22 possible symptoms, each on a scale from 0 to 6, where 0 means the patient is not experiencing that particular symptom and 6 means the symptom is most severe.

The symptom evaluation portion of the SCAT 3 is useful in the management of concussion in several ways. First, symptom inventories can be used to help diagnose a concussion in cases that are not clear. Fortunately, most athletes, when they are uninjured, are symptom free; they do not typically have any of the problems on the symptom evaluation portion of the SCAT 3. Therefore, if they sustain a blow to the head, followed by the symptoms listed on the evaluation, they would be diagnosed with a concussion. Some athletes, however, do experience headaches, difficulty concentrating, nausea, or other symptoms listed on the symptom scale even when they are uninjured. If the either number of symptoms they are experiencing or the intensity of their symptoms increase after a blow to the head, they might be diagnosed with a concussion. For this reason, many sports programs obtain baseline symptom inventories on athletes prior to the start of the athletic season, before the athletes are at risk of sustaining sport-related concussions.

Second, symptom inventories allow athletic trainers and doctors to determine which symptoms are bothering the athletes the most. Therefore, when therapies are started, they often are aimed at reducing the symptoms that are bothering the athletes most intensely. Furthermore, when athletes have prolonged recoveries that last several weeks, the symptom evaluation can be reviewed at each visit as a way of monitoring recovery. As the total score on the symptom evaluation decreases, athletes can see the progress as a sign of recovery, despite the fact that they are not yet fully symptom free. Last, if the score is increasing at any point or remaining stable for prolonged periods of time, consideration should be given to other therapies or perhaps other causes of the patient's symptoms.

Balance can also be affected by concussion. Concussion can result in difficulty with balance and unsteady walking. Balance can be assessed in multiple ways, some of which involve high-tech computerized machinery. In the setting of sports, during which concussions occur relatively commonly, balance is often assessed using something called the balance error scoring system (BESS). In order to perform the BESS, an athlete is placed in three stances: the double leg stance, single leg stance, and the tandem stance. The double leg stance consists of athletes standing with their feet together, side by side, such that they are touching. In the single leg stance, athletes stand on their nondominant foot. In the tandem stance, athletes stand with their feet heel to toe, with the nondominant foot in the back. In each of these stances, athletes undergo a 20-second trial during which they are asked to remain with their feet in the appropriate stance, their hands on their hips, and their eyes closed. An error occurs anytime when athletes lift their hands off of their hips, open their eyes, step, stumble or fall, bend their hips sideways or flex their hips forward more than 30 percent, lift a part of their feet off the ground, or remain out of the test position for more than 5 seconds. The number of errors made by the athlete is recorded.

The maximum amount of errors for a 20-second trial is 10. Originally, the BESS was performed once on the floor and once on a foam pad. This method is still recommended; however, a modified version is also used by only performing the trials on the floor.

Because the ability to balance varies among athletes, doctors, athletic trainers, and other medical professionals who care for athletes regularly will often measure balance before the start of an athletic season, in order to establish a baseline measure. This is important, because without a baseline measure it can be hard to know whether an athlete's balance has been affected by a concussion. For example, suppose a football player sustains a concussion and you, as his athletic trainer, are trying to tell whether he is recovered. You measure his BESS and he scores a 5. This could be a normal score for him, or it could be a sign of poorer than normal balance. If you know his BESS score was a 2 before the season, you would suspect that he is not yet recovered from his concussion. If you know his score was a 5 before the season, you feel confident that this score was reflective of his usual balance, when uninjured.

In another example, you might be evaluating a figure skater who had previously fallen on the ice and struck her head. She may score a 3 on her BESS. Because a 3 is an excellent score, you might suspect she has recovered from her concussion and clear her to return to skating. She may, however, simply have impeccable balance, as many figure skaters do. If she were tested at the beginning of the season, before she was injured, she may have scored a 0. If you do not have a baseline score, the BESS score can be difficult to interpret.

Cognition can also be affected by a concussion. The term cognition refers to conscious, intellectual activity. Cognitive activities are those activities that involve thinking, learning, remembering, concentrating, understanding, and reasoning. They are the activities required of students when they are doing their school work, such as reading or solving math problems. Many people perform cognitive activities just for fun. Some examples of cognitive activities that are commonly performed for fun include reading, playing video games, doing crossword puzzles, learning to play a musical instrument, and playing card games or board games such as chess. Since the brain cannot function properly after a concussion, these cognitive activities become more difficult. Recall that after a concussion, the brain requires more ATP to help it heal, to help pump sodium back out of the brain cells. Unfortunately, there is less ATP available because blood flow to the brain decreases after a concussion.

Typically, athletes with concussions have poorer memory when they are injured than they do prior to their injury. In addition, their reaction time is slower when they are suffering from a concussion. The speed at which they are able to think, to process information, is also decreased. Therefore, it takes athletes with a concussion longer to perform cognitive activities than when they are uninjured; things that normally they could do quite quickly, require additional time and effort. Clinicians often monitor the cognitive activity of athletes as a way of monitoring their recovery.

There are multiple ways of measuring cognitive function. Some common, standard ways may be familiar to students. I am sure many readers have had their ability to concentrate assessed by being asked to subtract serial 7s from 100. Classically, the examiner asks the person being examined to subtract 7 from 100, then subtract 7 from the answer, then subtract 7 from that answer, and so on. Each time, the person being examined states the answer out loud: 93, 86, 79, 72, and so forth. Another common test is to ask athletes suspected of having sustained a concussion to recite the months of the year backwards. These are some basic ways of measuring cognitive function. There are, however, much more thorough ways of measuring cognitive function. Some medical specialists known as neuropsychologists spend their careers measuring the cognitive function, interpreting the measurements, helping to determine the cause of any difficulties with cognition, and assist in the care of patients with poor cognitive function. Neuropsychological tests and neuropsychologists are often used in assessing concussions.

These traditional neuropsychological evaluations, however, can be time consuming often taking several hours to several days to complete. Furthermore, traditional assessments require that neuropsychologists are available to evaluate all the patients who need them. In an effort to make cognitive assessments more convenient to administer to athletes in particular, computerized versions have been developed in recent years. There are several advantages to computerized assessments. First, they can be administered to multiple athletes simultaneously in a relatively easy way. In addition, computerized programs have the ability to measure reaction time to 1/1,000 of a second, which is much more precise than an examiner with a stopwatch is able to do accurately. Finally, they allow for easy storage and rapid transfer of results among clinicians treating athletes that sustain sport-related concussions. Although this technology is relatively new, its use is increasing, particularly among athletes who have medical staff available to them, such as athletic trainers.

There are also, however, some downsides to computerized assessments. First, since they are relatively new, there is limited experience with them when compared to more traditional assessments. Second, they are not as thorough or complete as traditional assessments. Third, although they can measure cognitive function, they cannot interpret the assessments. In other words, they cannot give insight into why a given athlete scores a certain way. Cognitive tests can be affected by other reasons than concussion. Say, for example, a rugby player performs poorly on a computerized cognitive assessment. Yes, it may be because he has a concussion. It could also be, however, that he just broke up with girlfriend, was depressed about it, and was up all night thinking about it. His scores are likely to be poor because he is sad, tired, and not motivated to try very hard. He may be sick, dehydrated, distracted by an emotionally stressful situation in his life, all of which can affect his performance on these assessments. The computerized versions of these assessments only reveal his scores. With the traditional evaluation, the neuropsychologist can investigate and discover reasons for the scores, determining which factors may be affecting performance. Finally, computerized assessments can be administered by people who have not necessarily properly trained on them. Some may purchase the software, without taking the training on how to properly interpret them. This increases the risk that the scores will be improperly interpreted.

As with balance, cognition varies widely among athletes. Some athletes have impeccable memories, brisk reaction times, and fast processing speeds. Other athletes have difficulty with remembering things, slower reaction times, and take a relatively long time to process information. Thus, in an ideal situation, all athletes at risk of sustaining a concussion will have their cognitive function measured prior to the start of the season. These baseline measurements can be compared to scores measured after a concussion occurs, in order to help diagnose an injury in unclear situations and in order to monitor recovery. As with balance assessments, cognitive tests can be difficult to interpret without a baseline.

More recently, other assessments have been proposed that assess the ability of the eyes to move rapidly back and forth, which also can be affected by a concussion. Tests have been developed that assess the rapid eye movements of athletes before and after a concussion, as a means of both diagnosing and monitoring recovery from concussion. Others have used simple measures of reaction time by dropping a stick through the open hand of an athlete and asking the athlete to grasp the stick as fast as they can once it is released by the examiner. Nearly every year, multiple new methods for assessing concussion are being proposed in the medical literature and the marketplace. By the time this book is published, there will likely be dozens of additional assessments available.

Since concussion is largely a problem of brain function as opposed to a structural injury, there is currently no available means of "seeing" it or imaging it. By structural injury, I mean damage to the tissue itself.

Common structural injuries that readers may be familiar with are bruises, cuts, scrapes, and fractures. These injuries result in direct damage to body tissue or bone, and such damage can be seen either by looking at the skin or by getting an X-ray of the bone. There are images of the brain available, similar to X-rays, that allow doctors to see the tissue of the brain itself. Some of the more common ones are computed tomography (CT) and magnetic resonance images (MRIs). Since the problem with the brain that has a concussion is that it does not function properly, there is no structural damage. Therefore, concussion cannot be seen on CTs or MRIs. Concussion itself does not result in bruising, bleeding, rupturing, fracturing, or lacerating the brain. The brain is structurally intact, but is not functioning properly. Thus, modern-day imaging cannot identify concussion. There are some experimental methods for imaging the brain after concussion that are being tested now and may prove useful in the future. At the time of this writing, however, their utility remains experimental.

Ultimately, the diagnosis of concussion is based mainly on the medical history and the physical examination. The medical history is what a patient reports to the doctor about the injury. The classic history for a sport-related concussion involves some trauma to the head that led to the signs and symptom of concussion. A typical medical history from a patient would be:

> I was playing ice hockey a few days ago. I lost control of the puck as I was skating into the offensive zone. I looked down as I tried to regain control of the puck and this big defensemen body checked me, hitting me in the head with his shoulder. I fell backward and struck my head against the ice. I felt horrible. I had trouble skating off the ice, and felt like I was losing my balance. My teammates helped me off and took me to the athletic trainer. I was nauseous, had a headache, and felt like I was in a fog. My trainer says I kept asking him what we were doing there and who we were playing, which is weird, because it was the biggest game of the season. In any case, he took me out of the game. He told me to get lots of rest, stay home from practice, and check in with him by phone. Over the last few days, I have started to feel a lot better. But I still have headaches and the light bothers my eyes.

From the medical history, a doctor knows that the athlete has sustained trauma to the head followed by at least one sign of concussion, repetitive questioning, and some typical symptoms of concussion, headaches, nausea, and sensitivity to light. But these symptoms can also be caused by other injuries and medical conditions, including other head injuries. Therefore, after hearing the medical history, the doctor will perform a physical examination, which usually will include the assessment of brain functions. This examination will look for signs of injuries other than concussion, in order to ensure the athlete has no additional, and perhaps more emergent, injuries. Often, this examination will be followed by the specific measures of symptoms, balance, and cognitive function discussed previously. Sometimes, a picture of the brain such as a CT or MRI may be ordered to make sure there is not some other injury such as bleeding in the brain, although this is usually not necessary. Ultimately, an athlete who has sustained a blow to the head followed by the signs and symptoms of a concussion without the signs and symptoms of other injuries is diagnosed with a concussion. The signs and symptoms are often assessed by the medical history, physical examination, symptom inventories, balance assessments, and measures of cognition.

Please note that although I have discussed some specific assessments in this chapter, such as the SCAT 3, there are many assessments available, including symptom inventories, cognitive assessments, sideline assessments, and balance assessments, among others. Many have been well studied and validated for use in athletes at risk for sport-related concussion, others have not. The decision, as to which tests to use and when, is best left up to the treating clinician managing a given athlete's concussion.

Summary

Since concussion is a disturbance of brain function, albeit temporary, the best way to diagnose and monitor concussion is to assess brain function, often by assessing the three main domains in particular: symptom level, balance stability, and cognitive function. As athletes are at risk for concussions, medical providers caring for athletes often use standard measurements for each of these domains. Since symptom level, balance, and cognitive function can vary among uninjured athletes, baseline measurements obtained before the season starts are useful for comparison to assessments made after injury. The diagnosis of concussion is made by conducting a medical history, a physical examination, a symptom inventory, a balance assessments, and measures of cognitive function.

CHAPTER 6

Treatment and Management

The management of concussion varies depending on the stage of injury. In general, there are four main stages: baseline, acute, subacute, and prolonged. Baseline refers to the planning for a concussion prior to the start of the season, prior to athletes being at risk for concussion; acute refers to the first few moments and first few days after the injury occurs; subacute refers to the days and weeks after injury occurs; and prolonged refers to concussion symptoms which last longer than a month. Each of these stages is discussed further below.

BASELINE

All athletes who plan to participate in organized sports are encouraged to undergo a standard Preparticipation Physical Evaluation that has been developed by several medical societies, including the American Academy of Family Physicians, the American Academy of Pediatrics, the American Orthopaedic Society for Sports Medicine, and the American Osteopathic Academy of Sports Medicine. While the Preparticipation Physical Evaluation encompasses much more than just concussion, it does have components that specifically help in the evaluation of concussion and asks specifically about previous concussions athletes have sustained.

As mentioned previously, athletes are at particular risk of sustaining concussions, as it is a common injury in sports, accounting for approximately 13 percent of all injury sustained by high school athletes. Since athletic trainers, team physicians, parents, coaches, and athletes themselves are aware of this risk, baseline measurements of the areas of brain function most often affected by concussion are made. In the unfortunate event of a sport-related concussion, repeat measurements of the brain functions can be made and compared to the preinjury baseline measurements. These measurements can be used to help make the diagnosis of concussion in unclear cases, and to monitor recovery from concussion. Typically, baseline assessments are made of symptoms that are associated with concussion, balance, and cognition, as discussed in Chapter 3. Common concussion symptom inventories are Post-Concussion Symptom Inventory, the Rivermead Post-Concussion Symptoms Questionnaire, the British Columbia Post-Concussions Symptom Inventory, Graded Symptom Checklist, and the Post-Concussion Symptom Scale, among others. Some symptom inventories are incorporated into overall concussion assessment tools such as the Sport Concussion Assessment Tool version 3 (SCAT 3), Acute Concussion Evaluation (ACE), or the "Heads Up: Brain Injury in Your Practice" toolkit put out by the Centers for Disease Control and Prevention.

Balance is often measured by the Balance Error Scoring System discussed in Chapter 3, but there are others ways of doing it. Some devices use force plates, flat surface instruments that measure ground reaction forces between the feet and ground while an athlete is standing on or running across them, to assess balance. Others use video technology to gather information about the sway of the body. Some use accelerometers, which measure the acceleration of a body in motion. Some use a combination of these and other technologies to measure balance. Examples of such devices include Biodex Balance Assessment, Equilibrate, Neurocom, and the C3 Logix System, among others. Given the diverse capabilities and easy accessibility, modern-day smartphones and tablets are currently being explored as new technologies with the potential for measuring balance.

Cognition can be measured either by traditional neuropsychological assessments performed by a neuropsychologist. Such common assessments that have been used for assessing sport-related concussions include the Hopkins Verbal Learning Test, Trail Making Test Part B, Stroop Color and Word Test, Paced Auditory Serial Addition Test, Controlled Word Association Test, Symbol Digit Modalities Test, and the Color–Word Test, among others. These tests allow the examiner to measure different components of brain function including memory, reaction time, processing speed (the amount of time it takes to process information and arrive at an answer), concentration, and inhibition (the ability to inhibit an overlearned response). To give an example as to how these tests work, we will take a closer look at the Stroop Color and Word Test.

The Stroop Color and Word Test consists of three pages. On the first page, the words of various colors are printed in black ink. The examinee reads the words as quickly as possible, while being timed by the examiner. On the second page, there are "Xs" printed in colored ink. The examinee calls out the ink colors as quickly as possible, again while being timed by the examiner. On the third page is printed the words of various colors printed in a colored ink, but the color ink does not match the color of the word. The examinee must name the color ink in which a word is printed, while ignoring the actual word itself. For example, when faced with the word "Blue" in red ink, the examinee would answer correctly by saying "red."

As discussed in Chapter 3, there are computerized assessments of cognitive function, as well. These are computer-based tests similar to those listed in the previous paragraph. They are typically administered by an athletic trainer or a team physician. Some common available computerized assessments include ImPACT, Axon Sports, Concussion Resolution Index, Concussion Vital Signs, Computerized Cognitive Assessment Tool, XLNTbrain Sport, and Automated Neuropsychological Assessment Metrics.

ACUTE

The acute management of concussion occurs in the first few moments and days after injury. Concussions that occur during sports are usually due to a direct blow to the head. Please recall, however, that concussion results from rapid rotation or spinning of the brain and, therefore, direct blow to the head is not necessary in order for athletes to suffer concussions. Certainly, a direct blow to the head is the most common mechanism by which a concussion is sustained in sports. If an athlete is suspected of sustaining a concussion, medical personnel should be notified. Ideally, there will be an athletic trainer, emergency medical technician, or a physician on the sidelines who can respond immediately. The medical priorities are similar to those involved in any emergent situation. The responding medical provider should ensure that the athlete is breathing and has a beating heart. This is particularly important if the athlete is unconscious and not responding to questions. While concussion can result in a loss of consciousness (between 5% and 10% of sport-related concussions involve a loss of consciousness), it usually does not. Therefore, the medical staff must make sure there are no other conditions causing the athletes problems.

If the athlete is awake, medical staff must assess for all possible injuries. Any injury that could result in permanent disability or death must be quickly addressed and stabilized. The evaluation for concussion should occur only after it has been determined there are no emergent medical problems. Blows to the head can cause cervical spine injuries in addition to concussions. Therefore, an athlete suspected of having sustained a concussion should also be evaluated for a possible cervical spine injury.

Most of the time, concussion is much more subtle and occurs without a loss consciousness. In fact, concussions can be so subtle that they go unrecognized by other athletes, coaches, parents, referees, and medical staff. In addition, studies suggest that in some sports, only half of the athletes that sustain sport-related concussions report their injuries. Therefore, it is up to coaches, parents, medical staff, teammates, and other people who regularly attend sporting events to learn the signs and symptoms of concussion and alert the appropriate officials when they suspect an athlete has sustained a concussion.

Once a diagnosis of concussion is made, treatment consists initially of rest. There are two forms of rest used in the management of concussion early on. The first is physical rest. This is understood by most athletes. Although exercising and training is an important part of athletics, doing so in the setting of a concussion can increase an athlete's symptoms and, perhaps, prolong their recovery. Therefore, during the first few days after a concussion has occurred, athletes restrict their exercise, limiting the amount that they do, especially vigorous exercise such as bicycling, running, resistance training, weightlifting, and similar forms of exercise. In addition, athletes are instructed to avoid activities that place them at increased risk of blow to the head, even if they do not involve vigorous exercise, such as contact or collision sports participation or other risky activities, such as downhill skiing, mountain bicycling, among others.

The second form of rest is referred to as cognitive rest. As with exercise, intense cognitive activities that involve learning, remembering, thinking, and reasoning can result in an increase in symptoms and may prolong recovery, especially early on in the recovery process. Therefore, for the first few days after a concussion occurs, the athlete is asked to undergo cognitive rest—avoid activities that involve a lot of reasoning, thinking, concentrating, and memorizing. Such activities include schoolwork, reading, playing video games, playing cards or board games, and other similar activities.

In many cases, the symptoms from a sport-related concussion resolve quickly, after a matter of a few days, and therefore, cognitive and physical rest are often the only therapies that are necessary.

SUBACUTE

For some athletes, the symptoms of concussion last longer than a few days. Their recovery lasts into the subacute period, which begins after the first few days following injury and extends through the first four weeks. Hopefully, these athletes used cognitive and physical rest during the first few days after injury to speed their recovery. There is some emerging evidence, however, that after the first few days, continuing to restrict cognitive activity can result in a longer recovery. Therefore, after a few days of cognitive rest, athletes, particularly student athletes, are encouraged to start returning to their schoolwork gradually. Many athletes are able to maintain a full course load, complete all assignments, take all tests, and take all quizzes. Those who are able to do so should be allowed to. Some athletes, however, have such a slow processing speed and difficulty with memory that it is not possible for them to take their entire course load and maintain their grades at their current level. For these athletes, academic accommodations are given. Academic accommodations are adjustments and modifications made to a student's curriculum to help compensate for the disadvantages caused by the concussion. For example, since concussion can cause a slower processing speed, it can be harder for students with a concussion to finish tests in the same time allotted to uninjured students. Thus, students recovering from a concussion may be given extra time to complete tests and homework assignments. Some students with concussions might limit their schedules, taking only two or three courses until their recovery is complete. This is beneficial to the athletes, as it allows them to continue performing some of their schoolwork, maintain their grades at the current level, and avoid intense worsening of their symptoms. There are downsides to limiting the schedule to two or three courses, though. As the athlete recovers, the homework, test, quizzes, papers, and other assignments in the courses that the athlete is not keeping up in accumulate. Thus, when they recover fully, athletes with limited schedules often have fairly large amounts of work they need to make up. This can result in emotional stress, difficulty sleeping, and a decrease in grades, as the missed work has to be made up while the student continues to perform the ongoing work for current classes. It is best to try and strike a balance, where students with a concussion are completing as much homework as possible without their grades or their symptoms getting markedly worse. This gradual return to cognitive activity as tolerated usually begins after three to five days of cognitive rest.

Physical activity, particularly intense physical activity, is restricted for several days or weeks after injury, as it often results in worsening of symptoms and may prolong recovery. As with cognitive activity, however, there are some studies that suggest that introducing some low-risk physical activity may be not only safe, but also beneficial to recovery from concussion. Therefore, after an initial period of physical rest, athletes often start to engage in light aerobic activity, while staying below level of activity which exacerbates their symptoms.

PROLONGED

For a small percentage, somewhere between 2 and 3 percent, of athletes that sustain a sport-related concussion, their concussion symptoms last longer than a month. This is frustrating for the athletes, since they are not allowed to participate in the sports they enjoy. Furthermore, those athletes with academic accommodations may not be accomplishing much of their schoolwork. As they fall behind in school, they become anxious about how difficult it will be to make up work when they are better. This anxiety combined with the lack of exercise often results in poor sleep, with both trouble falling asleep and trouble staying asleep. Combine this poor sleep with a lack of exercise, and many of these athletes will have decreased energy during the day. All these effects, combined with the headaches that are so common after a concussion, can cause difficulty with concentration and memory. As you can see, prolonged recovery from concussion is frustrating. Furthermore, some of the therapies that are helpful shortly after the concussion, like physical and cognitive rest, can have undesirable effects as recovery becomes prolonged.

Therefore, if athletes with a concussion have not had a substantial improvement in their symptoms after the first few weeks of recovery, then additional therapies and changes to their management should be considered. As noted previously, after an initial rest period, light aerobic activity is safe and may improve recovery. Thus, some light exercise is often considered. This exercise often improves their mood, increases their daytime energy, and helps them sleep better.

Headaches can be treated with medication. As the headaches associated with concussion usually occur daily, many athletes are offered a preventative headache medication, a medication that is taken every day, at the same time, in order to prevent headaches from occurring. Whether or not a medication should be started and, if so, which medication, depends on many factors. Therefore, all decision, including the use of over-the-counter medications, should be discussed with the doctor treating the concussion.

Sleep can also be treated, initially with what is known as sleep hygiene. Most people nowadays are surrounded by constant stimulation from cell phones, computers, television, video games, and other electronic devices, often kept in the bedroom during sleep. Eliminating these devices from the bedroom and lying down to rest in a quiet, dark room may improve sleep quality.

Simply turning off these devices is not as effective as eliminating them from the room, as the mere presence of a computer, or for that matter a textbook or calendar, can often trigger stress and anxiety regarding the tasks of the following day, particularly for athletes who are often competitive, highly motivated people. Athletes with concussion can also improve their sleep by avoiding chemicals that increase alertness such as caffeine, nicotine and other chemicals found in tobacco products, energy drinks, and many sodas. If, after introducing these measures, athletes are still having difficulty sleeping, medications that help improve sleep may be considered.

While academic accommodations often allow students with concussions to resume school and maintain their grades, sometimes accommodations alone are not enough. In those situations, there are medications that may help improve concentration, memory, and mood of students with concussions that may be considered. Many of these medications are still experimental and not approved by the federal drug administration for the treatment of concussion. Therefore, they should only be prescribed by a doctor who is experienced and knowledgeable in the management of concussion.

Some athletes experience predominantly vestibular symptoms after a concussion. The vestibular system consists of parts of the ear and brain that help control balance, eye movements, and coordination. Vestibular symptoms are those that affect the vestibular system. Common vestibular symptoms that can occur after a concussion are dizziness, poor balance, vision problems such as blurry or double vision, or vertigo, which is a sensation of spinning. These symptoms can be addressed by a specific form of physical therapy, known as vestibular therapy, which can help alleviate these symptoms.

For some athletes, particularly those who have had major restrictions placed on their activities, who have sustained multiple injuries in a short time period, or who are in the midst of a long recovery, understandably develop other symptoms unrelated to the concussion. It is not uncommon for athletes with a concussion to stop exercising. This lack of exercise can result in decreased energy, trouble falling asleep at night, dizziness, depressed mood, irritability, and other symptoms. Athletes who miss school or some school assignments during recovery from their concussions will often suffer emotional stress as they fall behind in their schoolwork. This emotional stress can lead to difficulties sleeping at night, headaches, low energy, among other symptoms. One of the reasons athletes will often start safe, low-risk forms of exercise and a gradual return to their schoolwork after the first few days of initial rest is to avoid these complications. If easing these restrictions and allowing for a gradual return to safe activities isn't enough to alleviate emotional stress, however, counseling with sports psychologists or other professionals can help an athlete decrease symptoms and cope with the situation.

In addition, some athletes will sustain other injuries, such as neck muscle strain, at the time of their concussion. Neck muscle strains can also be associated with headaches. Thus, treating the co-occurring injuries may help resolve some symptoms.

RETURN-TO-PLAY

Athletes are considered recovered from their concussions when they no longer have symptoms from their injury and their balance and cognitive functions have returned to baseline. Once recovered, athletes can gradually start returning to their sports. First, student athletes will make up any missed schoolwork. They will then advance their physical exercise, according to guidelines published by international experts on sport-related concussion, beginning with light aerobic activity and advancing through specific stages to eventual game play.

Stage	Description of activity
1	No activity, complete rest. Proceed to level 2 once symptoms resolve.
2	Light aerobic exercise such as walking or stationary cycling.
3	Sport-specific exercise, such as skating for hockey players, running and dribbling for soccer and basketball players, and more, in addition to light resistance training.
4	Noncontact training drills and increased resistance training.
5	Full contact practices after receiving medical clearance from a doctor.
6	Game play.

If symptoms recur at any stage, exertion should stop for 24 hours. The next day, the athlete may resume exercise at the stage at which they previously had no symptoms. As noted previously, new evidence suggests that it may be safe, even beneficial, to start returning to low-risk activity even prior to full symptom resolution. Thus, some may start exercising before their symptoms have fully resolved, although they should be sure to avoid exercises that place them at risk for trauma to the head.

Summary

There are four main stages of concussion management: baseline, acute, subacute, and prolonged.

During the baseline stage, data is gathered on athletes while they are uninjured. This baseline data can be used to compare the performance after a concussion or suspected concussion occurs. Typical baseline evaluations include a Preparticipation Physical Evaluation, a symptom inventory, an assessment of balance, and an assessment of cognitive function, either traditional neuropsychological testing or a computerized cognitive assessment. The initial treatment of concussion, started during the acute stage, consists of physical and cognitive rest. Often, since most athlete recover quickly, this is the only treatment that is needed. For athletes whose recoveries continue into the subacute phase, a gradual increase in cognitive activity is recommended and academic accommodations may be put in place to assist with schoolwork. For those athletes whose symptoms are prolonged, light aerobic physical activity is safe and may be helpful in recovery. Sleep hygiene is used to improve sleep quality. For some athletes, medication to treat headaches, sleep disturbance, and other symptoms may be considered. Once an athlete has recovered completely, a gradual return-to-play protocol is used to return athletes to their sports safely.

CHAPTER 7

Prevention

Given the increased concern regarding concussions and the potential for long-term cumulative effects, the limited ability to definitively diagnose or determine recovery from concussion, and the limited number of therapies for concussion, it is not surprising that efforts are starting to turn toward the prevention of sport-related concussions. In an ideal world, we would be able to prevent these injuries before they happen, and the need for definitive treatment would be obsolete. We do not, however, live in an ideal world. Still, there are substantial possibilities for reducing the risk of sport-related concussions. There are two ways to go about this. One is trying decrease the risk of secondary injuries. Athletes who have sustained a concussion in the past are at increased risk for sport-related concussions in the future. The risk is highest shortly after the injury. As athletes get further and further away from their injury, the risk of additional injury decreases. Furthermore, there is evidence from animal studies that suggests that increasing the time between concussions decreases the potential for long-term effects and consequences. There are also attempts to prevent primary injuries, initial concussions. The strategies used for preventing initial concussions differ from those designed to prevent secondary injuries.

EDUCATION

Concussions that occur during sports are often not reported by the athletes themselves. There are many reasons for this underreporting of concussions. Some athletes do not recognize their symptoms as attributable to a concussion that has just occurred, but rather attribute their symptoms to other things such as dehydration or fatigue. Others do not stop to think about what might be causing their symptoms. Still other athletes do not want to give up playing time as it might let down or disappoint their team, coach, or parents. Other athletes do not want to miss playing time as they are afraid they might lose their starting position to someone who steps in to fill the role while they are recovering. Others simply enjoy playing sports and do not want to be removed. By educating athletes about the symptoms of concussion, the hope is that reporting will increase. The more capable athletes are of recognizing their symptoms as attributable to a concussion, or concerning for possible concussion, the more likely they will be to report it to their coach, parent, athletic trainer, physician, or other possible adults. At least that is the hope. Furthermore, if athletes understand the risks involved with returning to sport before full recovery from concussion, they may be more likely to report their injuries and remove themselves from play, thereby decreasing the risk of any complicating secondary injuries such as second impact syndrome. Thus, efforts to educate young athletes have been taken up by many societies and institutions. One of the more commonly used sets of educational materials was developed by the Centers for Disease Control and Prevention and is known as "Heads Up: Concussion in Sports." Within this set of tools, there are separate collections of materials for athletes, coaches, parents, and other interested parties. Each is designed to deliver the most important information in a way that is interpretable to the reader. And, there is some emerging evidence that these educational efforts are helpful in that the proportion of athletes reporting their concussions is improving, although these gains seem to be slow.

LEGISLATION

Recently, all the 50 states in the United States have introduced legislation regarding the diagnosis and management of athletes who sustain sport-related concussions. Most of these laws specify who should be evaluating the athlete who has sustained a suspected concussion and what requirements should be met prior to considering a return-to-play. These laws are also designed to try and reduce secondary injury that might occur by returning an athlete to sport prior to full recovery. There have been several well-described cases of athletes returning to play prior to full resolution of concussion symptoms who have gone on to suffer devastating injuries.

EQUIPMENT

Equipment manufacturers have been actively pursuing equipment and technology that would reduce the risk of concussion. While many people believe helmets in sports like football and ice hockey were introduced in order to reduce the risk of concussion, they were in fact designed to prevent more devastating and even catastrophic brain injuries such as skull fractures and blood within the skull or within the brain tissue itself. Helmets are very effective at preventing skull fractures and blood in the brain. Therefore, helmets should be worn, properly fitted, and using all securing straps. Helmets were not, however, designed to reduce the incidence of concussion originally. Efforts are being made currently to try and develop helmets that will reduce the risk of sport-related concussion. Some studies have suggested there may be variability in the incidence of sport-related concussion, while others show that the type of helmet does not translate into a different risk of sustaining a concussion.

In addition to helmets, many companies are trying to develop mouth guards that will decrease the risk of concussion. Many concussions that occur during sports result from a direct blow to the chin of the athlete. Thus, the thought is that a mouth guard can be developed that would absorb most of that force, before it is transmitted to the skull and brain, and perhaps the risk of concussion could be reduced. There is some evidence suggesting that mouth guards may do this; however, the evidence is limited and has been criticized by many researchers and investigators.

PHYSICAL CONDITIONING

Concussion is caused by a rapid rotational acceleration, or spinning, of the brain. A force is applied to the skull resulting in this rapid acceleration. As many of you will know from your high school physics class, force is equal to mass times acceleration ($F = ma$). Therefore, for a given force, the greater the mass is, the lower the resulting acceleration. Thus, scientists thought that if you could increase the effective mass of the head, it would reduce the resultant acceleration after a collision of given force occurred. It would be difficult and potentially unsafe to simply increase the mass of the head by having athletes wear large, bulky, massive materials. One might, however, be able to more safely increase the effective mass of the head by having it attached more firmly to the rest of the athlete's body. The head is attached to the remainder of the athlete's body by the muscles of the neck. The more firmly the head is attached to the body, the more the head and the body will act as a single unit. If an athlete's muscles are relaxed, the head is less effectively attached to the rest of the body and, therefore, the effective mass of the head is relatively small. If, however, the athlete's muscles are contracted when the head is struck, the effective mass of the head comes closer to the mass of the head and body together, they are rigidly held together by the muscles of the neck and act as one unit.

Thus, some have argued that athletes who anticipate a collision and are therefore in a state of having their muscles flexed are at a reduced risk of sustaining a concussion. Indeed, preliminary evidence has demonstrated this phenomenon in ice hockey, American football, and other sports. One method discussed for reducing the risk of sport-related concussion, therefore, is what is known as collision anticipation. In youth sports in particular, athletes tend to follow the ball or hockey puck or other object that is the main focus of attention. When doing so, often athletes become so focused they will not look at their surroundings. One can imagine a scenario where multiple ice hockey players are heading into the boards behind the net trying to gain control of the puck. If one of those athletes is unaware of his surroundings, he might gain control of the puck and attempt to turn up ice only to be struck by an oncoming opponent. In such a circumstance, when he does not anticipate the collision being delivered by his opponent, his risk of concussion is great. If, however, we teach that same athlete to look around and be aware of his environment as he heads into the boards to gain control of the puck, he may see the oncoming opponent and brace himself for the pending collision. In such a circumstance, it might reduce his risk of injury. Therefore, education on how to anticipate collisions by coaches might decrease the risk of concussion.

For similar reasons, strengthening the muscles of the neck might decrease the risk of sport-related concussion. When muscles are being contracted as a means of firmly attaching the head to the remainder of the body and increasing the effective mass of the head in order to reduce the acceleration after a collision, the stronger the neck muscles are, the more capable they are of rigidly attaching the head to the body. Therefore, strengthening the muscles of the neck may also lead to decreased risk of concussion. Indeed, there is some preliminary data showing that athletes with stronger neck muscles have a lower incidence of concussion compared to their colleagues with weaker necks.

It should be noted here that some athletes, female athletes in particular, are reluctant to strengthen the muscles of the neck as they do not want to appear large and bulky. The increase in both size and mass of muscles in response to resistance training is dependent to a large degree on the presence of testosterone, a naturally occurring hormone. Testosterone is present at much greater levels in male athletes than in female athletes. Thus, female athletes tend not to become bulky and are, therefore, less likely to develop large bulky neck muscles in response to strengthening. They do, however, increase the strength of their muscles and are likely to reduce their risk of concussions as much as their male counterparts in response to a strength training regimen.

Last, and perhaps most importantly, changes of the rules of the game are likely to be the most effective means of reducing the risk of concussion in sports. By studying the circumstances surrounding the occurrence of concussions that occur during sports, researchers can determine what are the most high-risk activities and sports. This information can be used to decrease the occurrence of sport-related concussions by limiting or altering the rules such that the situations in which concussion most commonly occur are reduced. This might decrease the incidence of concussion. In ice hockey in particular, something known as fair play rules have been observed to decrease the risk of concussion. Most of the time, how successful a team is depends on its wins and losses. According to fair play rules, however, teams score points for keeping the number of penalty minutes they accrue at a minimum. Teams that accrue penalties at a greater rate lose points. These points factor into their overall standings. When fair play rules are used, penalties are decreased substantially and this decrease in penalties is associated with a decreased risk of injuries, including sport-related concussions.

SUMMARY

Sport-related concussions have become a much greater concern to athletes, parents, and coaches over the last decade or two. In response, efforts have been made to try and prevent concussions from occurring in sports. This is an ongoing area of research and investigation. Some of the methods, such as education and legislation, are designed to try and reduce the risk of secondary injuries that occur when athletes return to their sport prior to full recovery. Other methods, such as equipment, physical conditioning, and rule changes, are efforts to decrease the risk of primary injury, the initial concussions themselves. There is preliminary evidence suggesting that some strategies may be successful, but at present, the evidence is preliminary and it is difficult to make definitive conclusions as to which are most effective.

CHAPTER 8

The Cumulative Effects of Concussion

Fortunately, the symptoms of most concussions, particularly those caused during sports, resolve within a few days, with relatively few lasting longer than a month. Most often, symptoms are worse shortly after injury, and gradually improve over time. While symptoms can be exacerbated by periods of prolonged concentration and mental effort, or by periods of intense exercise, the overall course of symptoms should be a gradual decrease in intensity, decrease in frequency, and ultimately, resolution. Studies suggest that professional, collegiate, and high school athletes recover from their concussions quite readily. In a study of nearly 2,000 collegiate athletes, Guskiewicz and colleagues showed that nearly 90 percent of athletes recovered from their sport-related concussions within the first 10 days. Subsequent studies have shown similar findings. In multiple studies using data from an online injury surveillance system, Dawn Comstock and her colleagues have shown that more than 95 percent of athletes that sustain a concussion during high school sports have full resolution of their symptoms within a month.

Unfortunately, the Centers for Disease Control and Prevention estimates that there may be as many as 3.8 million sport-related traumatic brain injuries occurring each year, and the vast majority of these injuries are concussions. Thus, while only 2–3 percent of these athletes suffer prolonged symptoms, this small percentage represents a fairly large overall number of people. Many recent studies have tried to predict which athletes will suffer prolonged concussion as opposed to the relatively brief experience of most athletes. Factors that have been hypothesized as producing a long recovery include the age of the athlete at the time of injury, the sex of the athlete, whether or not the athlete experienced acute onset of dizziness, whether or not the athlete had amnesia, overall symptom level after injury, and the number of previous concussions.

Although the symptoms of concussions sustained during sports tend to be relatively short lived for most athletes, they do have a cumulative effect. That is to say, when an athlete has sustained a concussion of the brain, the injury leaves behind some effects that do not seem to resolve. Indeed, these effects are often small and do not affect the athlete in their daily life nor inhibit their ability to succeed in the future. In fact, the effect is so small that it is difficult for scientists and doctors to observe it. But many athletes return to their chosen sports after having sustained a concussion, and thus, they place themselves at risk for additional concussions. When they sustain additional concussions, the effects of their prior concussions can be observed. For example, athletes who have sustained previous concussions are more likely to lose consciousness with an additional injury than those who sustain a first concussion. Furthermore, the overall time to resolution of their symptoms seems to be longer, on average, if they have sustained prior concussions.

In a landmark study by a neuropsychologist named Dorothy Gronwall, patients who were sent to her clinic for evaluation of their cognitive function were separated into two groups, those who had sustained their first concussion and those who had sustained their second concussion. She noticed that those with their second injury performed worse on measures of information processing speed, calculation, and concentration, and that it took them longer to return to more typical levels of function than patients with their first injury.

Since then, there have been multiple other studies showing the cumulative effect of concussions, including those sustained during sports. Athletes who have sustained previous concussions are more likely to lose consciousness and suffer amnesia with additional concussions than athletes who sustain their first concussion. In addition, athletes who have sustained prior concussions have longer recoveries, more pronounced symptoms, and more pronounced examination findings with additional injuries than those athletes who sustain their first lifetime concussion.

More recently, researchers hypothesized that the concussions sustained during sports might have a delayed effect and cause problems for former athletes later in life. Early in the 20th century, some physicians described what they called Punch-Drunk Syndrome, which has since been termed by various names such as dementia pugilistic, traumatic encephalopathy, chronic traumatic brain injury, and more recently, chronic traumatic encephalopathy (CTE). Doctors noted that boxers, in particular those who were described as sluggers and had relatively long careers, suffered from problems later in life such as headaches, slurred speech, shuffling gait, and multiple other symptoms. They hypothesized that, perhaps, the blows they took to the head during their boxing career, and specifically the concussions they sustained during their boxing careers, led to those problems later in life. Since that time, the brains of some boxers, after they had passed away, were assessed by pathologists. Pathologists are doctors who study the body after death in order to determine the cause of death and other potentially contributing factors. Pathologists noted that there were abnormalities of the brains of these boxers. Specifically, the brains of these boxers appeared to have shrunk over time. The ventricles (holes in the middle of the brain where cerebrospinal fluid is made) appeared larger. And there were abnormal proteins in the brain, a deformed version of an essential protein, known as hyperphosphorylated cis tau. They hypothesized that the blows to the head sustained over years of boxing led to these changes in the brain, and that the changes in the brain were associated with the signs and symptoms noted by physicians later in some boxers' lives.

In the last few decades, similar findings have been reported among former professional football players. There have been multiple reports of football players, as well as soldiers, athletes in other sports, and others who sustained repetitive trauma to the head over their lifetime, and later in life developed emotional problems, headaches, difficulty with memory, who, at autopsy, were noted to have changes similar to the brain as those seen in the boxers previously described. This led to the hypothesis the concussions sustained during sports have a delayed effect, showing up years after sports participation had ceased in the form headaches, troubled memory, other symptoms potentially associated with the changes to the brain observed by these pathologists.

Since some of these athletes had never been diagnosed with a concussion, some researchers have hypothesized that maybe it is not only the concussions themselves, but also the multiple blows to the head sustained during sports that do not result in the signs and symptoms necessary to make diagnosis of concussion that may contribute to these effects. Thus, it has been suggested that these blows, known as subconcussive blows, have a cumulative effect that can cause problems later in life and may, in fact, be risk factors for the entity known as CTE. Furthermore, studies during a season of sports have noted that athletes participating in sports that involve repeated blows to the head, even those who have not been diagnosed with a concussion, have developed decreases in their cognitive function, increases in their overall symptoms, and changes in their brains that can be seen on magnetic resonance images. This has led to a discussion about the effects of subconcussive blows to the head sustained during sports and whether or not certain sports should be banned.

The evidence, however, is not fully clear. Some studies of former athletes with no history of concussion reveal similar quality of life in various domains between those at high risk for subconcussive blows such as collision sport athletes, who played sports like American football, rugby, and men's ice hockey where purposeful body-to-body collisions are part of the game, and noncollision, noncontact sport athletes who played sports where body-to-body blows are rare and unexpected if they occur at all, such as swimming, golf, tennis, and cross-country running. These studies seem to suggest that exposure to subconcussive blows in these sports is not associated with a difference in quality of life later in life, at least at the levels of and for the duration that most athletes are exposed.

SUMMARY

While most athletes will recover quickly from sport-related concussions, a small percentage will go on to have symptoms for a prolonged period. As concussions are common, this small percentage represents a large number of athletes. Those with prolonged recoveries may be treated with therapies to manage their most troublesome symptoms. Athletes who sustain one or two concussions in sports are not at significantly higher risk of long-term problems than the general population. Concussions can, however, have cumulative effects, leading to problems as more and more concussions are sustained. Some former athletes undergo changes to the brain believed to result from either the multiple concussions they sustained during their playing careers or the common subconcussive blows to the head associated with certain sports. These changes have been termed CTE. While concussions have been demonstrated to have a cumulative effect, the role of subconcussive blows in the development of CTE or other problems with the brain remains unclear.

CHAPTER 9

Managing Athletes with a Concerning Concussion History

Although most athletes who sustain a concussion during sports will recover quickly and have an uncomplicated course and the management of their injuries and return-to-play is relatively straightforward, there are situations where it is more complicated. As you can imagine, some athletes in the high-risk sports, particularly collision sports such as boxing, mixed martial arts, American football, men's ice hockey, rugby, men's lacrosse, and so forth, may sustain multiple concussions over their careers. As we just learned, concussions can have a cumulative effect. Therefore, the timing of return-to-play and even deciding whether or not to return these athletes to their chosen sports can be a difficult decision. In addition, some athletes will have prolonged recoveries, with symptoms lasting more than a month, which also may complicate their management and decisions regarding the return to sport. Other athletes will have pronounced symptoms or more substantial deficits in cognitive function that will factor into their management decisions regarding if and when to return them to play. Some athletes will seem to become more susceptible, seem to sustain concussions more easily, due to collisions of decreasing force. Still other athletes, after having sustained a concussion, will have some hesitancy about returning to their sports associated with anxiety and fear. This may be due to concerns over the potential for cumulative effects, or due to concerns over suffering an injury again and experiencing the same symptoms and dysfunction that they suffered with previous injuries. Furthermore, the overall goals of the athlete may affect these decisions; professional athletes who earn their living playing a sport may be willing to take additional risks that those who are playing just for fun and enjoy alternate, safer sports just as much, are not willing to take. All of these factors play a role in the decisions as to when and if to return athletes to their sports, particularly collision and contact sports, which carry a higher risk of concussion. Each of these complicating factors is discussed in this chapter.

MULTIPLE INJURIES

It is not uncommon, as noted above, for athletes to sustain more than one sport-related concussion. As we learned in previous chapters, the effects of concussion can be cumulative, that is to say, every time an athlete experiences a concussion it can leave some effect on the brain that does not resolve. While in most cases this effect is minor and is unlikely to affect the athlete in any perceptible way, as the number of concussions accumulates, the effects can become more pronounced. Therefore, when athletes sustain multiple concussions, they and their treating clinicians need to devote substantial consideration to whether or not they should return to their chosen sports. Furthermore, if the athlete chooses to go back to the given sport, consideration as to the timing of return-to-play must be considered. Unfortunately for athletes, parents, doctors, and other medical personnel, it is unknown how many concussions can be sustained before leading to perceptible effects. In fact, the answer to "how many concussions is too many?" likely varies between athletes, being different for each athlete. It may also vary by the severity of the concussions sustained, other coexisting medical conditions, and many other factors that we as researchers and doctors have not yet even considered. As you can see, the decision as to whether or not to return an athlete to a given sport can be complicated. Any such decision should be made in conjunction with a doctor who is well versed in the area of sport-related concussions. In general, the more concussions athletes sustain, the more difficult it is to return them to contact, collision, and combat sports.

As noted throughout this text, most athletes who sustain concussions during sports recover quite quickly, more than 95 percent within a month. There are, however, athletes who experience symptoms that last longer than a month. When such cases occur, particularly if the athletes have sustained more than one concussion all of which have resulted in symptoms lasting longer than a month, most clinicians are more hesitant to return the athletes to their sports. While it is true that those athletes who sustained prior concussions are more likely to have a prolonged period of symptoms than athletes who have experienced only one concussion, it is not absolutely consistent. Studies are done on populations as opposed to individuals. If you take 100 athletes who sustained their first lifetime concussion, the average duration of symptoms they experience is shorter than 100 athletes who sustained their second concussion or greater. For individuals, however, they may experience three or four weeks of symptoms after their first lifetime concussion and then have symptoms that resolve in the matter of a few days after their second lifetime concussion. Nonetheless, athletes who have experienced previous sport-related concussions are at higher risk of developing longer symptoms than those who have sustained their initial lifetime concussion. Therefore, athletes who have a medical history that includes a concussion with symptoms lasting for an unusually long period of time require a more in-depth evaluation when deciding when and if they should return to their chosen sports.

Fortunately, for most athletes who sustain a sport-related concussion, the symptoms are relatively mild. There are, however, athletes who sustain more profound symptoms that have a greater impact on their quality of life during the period of recovery. When athletes sustain more pronounced, bothersome, and worrisome symptoms after their concussion, particularly if they have sustained multiple concussions all of which have involved pronounced and debilitating symptoms, then the decision whether or not to return them to contact or collision sports involves more careful deliberation. Plus, while some athletes may experience only mild symptoms, the effects on their cognition during the period of recovery may be profound. It is well demonstrated in medical literature that athletes who sustain sport-related concussions can have decreases in their cognitive functioning, including difficulty with memory, difficulty concentrating and performing calculations, slowed ability to process information, and slowed reaction time, as well as other effects on cognitive functioning. If those effects are dramatic or substantial, particularly when athletes have sustained multiple injuries with substantial effects on their cognition, it is more difficult to return them to play.

Similarly, we have all seen collisions during sports that result in a concussion, and indeed, while viewing the collision, the viewers expect that such a major, high-force collision might result in concussion. There are, however, athletes who sustain concussions with a typical high-force collision, but as time goes on, they appear to sustain concussions more and more easily; even minor blows to the head that typically would not be expected to cause any symptoms or bother them seem to result in the signs and symptoms of concussion. When an athlete appears to be sustaining concussions with less and less force, clinicians managing these athletes become more concerned and have to think carefully as to whether or not it will be safe to return them to their chosen sports.

Finally, some athletes, after sustaining a sport-related concussion, develop anxiety and fear regarding the injury. Some have experienced a prolonged recovery, major symptoms, or profound deficits in their cognition after their sport-related concussions, and although they have recovered, they have a substantial amount of anxiety about the risk of additional injury. If their injury has negatively impacted their quality of life dramatically, it is quite understandable that they would be reluctant to put themselves at risk for additional concussions, and the potential to go through it all again. Still, other athletes may be concerned about the stories they read in the newspaper, see on the news, hear on the radio, or hear about when they are watching sports on television. They may be concerned that the concussions they sustain now will lead to problems later in life such as headaches, depression, mood swings, memory problems, or even an increased risk of suicide. These reports receive a lot of attention in the general press and, therefore, athletes who sustain concussions are understandably concerned about their own risk of developing problems later in life. These athletes may experience anxiety about their own injuries and about the possibility of future injuries. This anxiety, fear, emotional stress can have symptoms of its own. While we outlined in previous chapters that concussion itself can cause headaches, difficulties with sleep, low energy, and other symptoms, many of these symptoms can be caused by anxiety or emotional stress. One can imagine that athletes who sustain concussions and are worried about the potential for future effects on their memory, mood, and other medical problems might have difficulty sleeping at night. This lack of sleep may result in decreased energy during the day, increased risk of headaches, and many other symptoms. Sometimes, when an athlete experiences these symptoms shortly after a concussion, it can be difficult to tell which symptoms are due to the concussion and which are due to this anxiety and emotional stress. Obviously, it will be important for doctors to know the cause of the symptoms in order to treat them appropriately. In addition, once treated, suffering such anxiety, emotional stress, or depression after an injury must be considered when deciding when and if athletes should return to their chosen sports. Some of these athletes will become quite anxious again, even after minor blows to the head that are highly unlikely to result in concussion. It can be difficult to return to sports with such a high level of anxiety, as common blows to the head result in undue and unwarranted fear, decreased quality of life, and possibly symptoms, even in the absence of concussion. In such a situation, thought must be given to removing an athlete from sport or building in a longer symptom-free waiting period.

   In addition, the age of the athlete is a factor when considering returning the athlete to sports. The effects of concussion, including recovery times, potential for long-term problems, and other factors, may vary according to the age of the athlete. In addition, the goals of the athletes and their families may vary according to age. In fact, the timing of the injuries and the effects that they may have on later life problems may vary according to age. One can easily imagine that if a fifth grader sustains a concussion that affects her memory and ability to concentrate, she may have a decrease in academic performance. If the student was previously scoring mostly "As" in her coursework but is now experiencing difficulty with memory and concentration, she may have a drop in her grades and end up getting more Cs and Ds at the end of the semester. For a fifth grader, however, this decrease in academic performance is unlikely to affect her long-term future, so long as her grades improve back to their previous levels once she has recovered from her concussion. This is not necessarily true for older athletes. Many juniors in high school are preparing to apply to colleges. Many colleges focus closely on the academic performance of high school students during their junior and first semester of their senior years. Therefore, if juniors in high school sustain concussions that result in problems with memory and concentration, particularly if they last for prolonged periods, the resulting drops in their grades from mostly "As" and "Bs" down to "Cs" and "Ds" may have more consequential effects on their future. It may decrease their chances of getting into college, or at least the college of their choice. This may have effects on their future job prospects, among other things. It should be noted that in order to avoid this type of situation, doctors managing athletes with sport-related concussions ask for academic accommodations to be made that allow athletes to complete their coursework in a reasonable timeframe, while obtaining their previously demonstrated level of performance. In situations where, despite these accommodations, the grades do slip for the period of recovery, some doctors will write a letter to go along with the student athlete's college application explaining the situation during that time period. Still, it is unclear how colleges interpret such letters or how much of a difference they make in the application process.

Furthermore, many athletes are employed. One can imagine that if you are fatigued during the day, having difficulty sleeping at night, having headaches, have difficulty concentrating, and have problems with memory, this may affect your performance at work. Those struggling to complete their duties at work are less likely to advance to higher positions, to be promoted, and more likely to be reprimanded or even dismissed. Therefore, occupational accommodations are often requested by the doctors managing them, as long as it is appropriate. For professional athletes, this represents a dilemma. Many professional athletes, particularly those in contact, collision, or other high-risk sports, cannot perform their duties safely in the setting of recovery from a concussion and, therefore, cannot return to work. Many worry that this may jeopardize their standing on the team. Indeed, there have been athletes quoted in the media expressing their disappointment and frustration when they miss a game due to a concussion and another athlete steps into fill their position—and performs so well that even when the original athlete has recovered, the backup athlete continues in the starting position. Unfortunately, this has led some athletes to downplay their symptoms in order to avoid losing their position to someone currently on the bench.

Given all of these reasons, athletes, parents, their treating doctors, and other important people in the athletes' lives must consider the number of concussions the athletes have sustained over their lifetimes, the duration of symptoms they have suffered after each concussion, the severity of symptoms they have suffered after each concussion, the cognitive deficits experienced after their concussions, the degree of force required to produce their concussions, and the anxiety and emotional stress suffered by the athletes after their concussions, when considering whether or not to return them to their sports. In general, the greater the number of previous concussions, the longer the symptoms, the more severe the symptoms, the more pronounced the cognitive dysfunction, the increased fear and anxiety, or the lower the force necessary to produce injury, the more difficult it is to allow athletes to continue playing.

Even when athletes might be able to return to their sports safely, the timing of return-to-play is also a factor. Studies have demonstrated that athletes who sustain concussions in a short time period are more likely to have longer recoveries than those whose concussions are separated in time to a greater degree. Furthermore, animal studies suggest that animals that sustain concussions closer together in time are more likely to have long-term, permanent effects on their cognition than animals whose concussions are separated further in time. For these reasons, many clinicians recommend a symptom-free waiting period, even after athletes recover from their concussions. The symptom-free waiting period may vary according to other factors such as the age of the athlete, the sports to which they wish to return, the number of prior concussions, the overall goals of the athlete, and many other factors. It is possible, however, that the potential for long-term problems from multiple concussions may be reduced by spacing the injuries out over time, which involves removing the athlete from risk for longer periods of time than one otherwise might.

SUMMARY

The management of concussion can be complicated and may be modified by assessing many factors. When deciding when and if to return an athlete to sports, the overall number of concussions the athlete has sustained during his or her lifetime must be considered. The duration of recovery from each previous injury, the severity of symptoms after injury, the severity of cognitive dysfunction after injury, the resulting anxiety and fear after each injury, and the effect on quality of life must all be taken into consideration when considering whether or not to return athletes to their sports. Furthermore, if the concussions appear to be occurring with decreasing amounts of force, further consideration must be given to whether or not the athlete can safely return to his or her sport. If the decision is made to return the athlete to sport, any of these modifying or complicating factors may prompt the athlete and the clinician to consider a longer symptom-free waiting period. This symptom-free waiting period should not simply consist of waiting, but rather, during this symptom-free waiting period the athletes should train to become faster, stronger, more agile, and better at their sports. Preliminary data suggest that the greater the muscle strength of the neck and shoulders, the lower the risk of sustaining a concussion. Thus, athletes who are in a symptom-free waiting period should consider working with a physical therapist or personal trainer in order to safely strengthen the muscles of the neck and shoulder. Furthermore, sport-specific skills training that can be conducted without risk of a blow to the head should also be encouraged. The goal here is that, when the athletes return to sport, they will be faster, stronger, and more agile with stronger neck muscles, all in an effort to reduce their risk of sustaining additional concussions.

Finally, and perhaps most importantly, the ultimate goals of the athletes need to be considered when deciding whether or not to return athletes to their sports. One can imagine the situation is quite different depending on the athletes' situations. The young athlete—who is 15 years old, playing high school football, ultimately wants to become a veterinarian, is not particularly good at football, and would rather run cross country, a sport in which he excels—might decide the risks of participating in football, particularly after having sustained a sport-related concussion, outweigh the benefits of participating. This particular athlete might be able to get the benefits of sport by running cross country without the higher risk of sport-related concussion that comes with football. On the other hand, an athlete who is playing professional football, who spent his entire life training for football, is earning his living by playing football, supports his family by playing football, and afterwards plans to coach football, may derive much more substantial benefits from football and might choose to continue to play after a concussion, despite the risks. Obviously, over time, the risks involved in continuing to participate and the benefits involved in continuing to participate change and, therefore, the process of weighing the risks and benefits should be ongoing, repeated after various events such as additional injuries. The process of weighing the risks of participation in a given sport against the benefits should consider any injury, not just concussion. Although it gets much less attention, the risk of catastrophic injury, defined as death or permanent neurological damage, is much higher among male gymnasts than football players. As a result, many parents discourage their male children from participating in gymnastics. They have decided that the risks of catastrophic injury outweigh the potential benefits to their son and therefore encourage their son to participate in other sports. Still, other parents recognize that, while the risk of catastrophic injury is higher in gymnastics than any other team sports, it is still relatively low. They see the enjoyment their son gets out of participating in gymnastics, the improvement in his self-esteem, the friendships he has made, and how the tremendous physical activity and conditioning involved in gymnastics have made him healthy, strong, and confident. For them, the benefits of participating outweigh the risks and, therefore, they encourage their son to participate in gymnastics. The benefits vary between sports, and within a particular sport, they vary from athlete to athlete. The risks also vary between sports and within a given sport, vary from athlete to athlete. Therefore, this process should be undertaken carefully by people who are knowledgeable about the risks and benefits and should be made on a personal and individualized basis.

CHAPTER 10

Common Examples of Athletes Sustaining Concussions

While discussion in general terms is necessary and useful, examples illustrating the points discussed are often more useful and clear. Therefore, this chapter will go through some examples of athletes with concussions, illustrating how they are injured, diagnosed, and managed. Some of the athletes in these examples will have typical, quick, uncomplicated recoveries, while others will have more prolonged, complicated courses. Furthermore, these examples will illustrate the thought process when making decisions regarding whether or not athletes should return to their chosen sports and, if they do return to their sports, how the timing of their return is considered.

EXAMPLE 1: TYPICAL RECOVERY

Connor plays for his high school lacrosse team. He is one of the most skilled players on the team, and last year led the team in goals. It is now preseason and Connor's athletic trainer is preparing the team for the event of possible injuries. As such, he is collecting baseline data from athletes. Connor is called to the athletic trainer's office. He sits down quietly and alone in a room where he is given a list of symptoms followed by a numbered scale from zero, meaning he does not have that symptom at all, to six, meaning that he suffers that symptom quite severely. On this scale, Connor ranks all the symptoms he is currently experiencing. As he is healthy, uninjured, and fortunate enough not have any medical conditions, Connor circles zero for all of the included symptoms. Once he is finished, he emerges from the athletic training room. His athletic trainers sit him down at a computer, once again alone in a quiet space, and log him into a baseline neurocognitive assessment. Connor enters some background information into the system and then is given puzzles, games, and other tests of his memory, his ability to concentrate, the speed with which he thinks, and his reaction time. All in all, it takes Connor approximately 30 minutes to complete this assessment. Once he is finished, he again emerges from the room to visit his athletic trainer. His athletic trainer then takes out a stopwatch and puts Connor in various positions, both on the surface of the athletic training room and then on an enlarged piece of foam. He is asked to hold each position with his eyes closed for a total of 20 seconds. His athletic trainer records the number of errors he makes, if any, during each 20-second period. All this information is placed in a folder with Connor's name.

The following day, during preseason workouts, Connor's athletic trainer calls him off the field and tells him it is time for him to get his sideline assessment. He is pulled from play in the middle of the practice, so he is tired, sweaty, and somewhat dehydrated, simulating the circumstances he might be in when he sustains a suspected concussion during a lacrosse practice or game. On the sidelines, he is asked a series of questions designed to test his ability to think and concentrate, his memory, and his orientation. All this information is recorded by the athletic trainer and once again placed in Connor's medical folder. All the members of the lacrosse team are put through the same baseline assessments.

As the season continues, Connor once again has an excellent showing. He is leading the league in assists and is second to only one other player on his team with regards to goals scored. There is even talk about Connor being chosen as the current year's (2016) captain.

One Saturday, Connor and his teammates are playing their archrivals. The game is nearing the end of the second half. The other team has a man in the penalty box and, therefore, Connor's team is executing their extra man offense plays. Connor receives a pass from his teammate which is slightly off the mark, causing him to lunge for the pass. As he does so, he is struck by a much larger defenseman who is about 4 inches taller and 25 pounds heavier than Connor. The defenseman's shoulder strikes Connor in the head. He falls to the ground and remains down for approximately 5 seconds. As he stands up, he is visibly off-balance. He is escorted to the sidelines and one of his teammates brings him to his athletic trainer. There, Connor reports that he has a headache, feels a little bit nauseous, and is having some ringing in his ears, in addition to feeling dizzy and unsteady on his feet. His athletic trainer performs a series of tests as part of the physical examination. Ultimately, he tells Connor that he has sustained a sport-related concussion and puts him on the bench.

Every few minutes or so, the athletic trainer returns to Connor and reexamines him, asking a series of additional questions. When the game is over, the athletic trainer lets Connor's parents know what happened and recommends that they keep an eye on him that evening and report any unusual behavior or any concerning findings to Connor's pediatrician. Connor is instructed not to engage in vigorous exercise for the next few days and to avoid large amounts of mental exertion. Connor is specifically instructed to avoid reading, playing video games, and doing his homework for the next few days, after which time he should return to his athletic trainer.

Connor goes home with his parents and follows the instructions. Fortunately, he continues to improve Saturday evening and all day Sunday. When he wakes up Monday morning, he is feeling markedly better, although he still has a slight headache and perhaps a slight feeling of dizziness. He goes to school and after his classes he reports to his athletic trainer. That Wednesday, four days after his injury, Connor reports to his athletic trainer that he is completely back to normal. His athletic trainer starts him working on a stationary bicycle, which goes quite well. After 20 minutes on the bicycle, Connor still has no headaches, no dizziness, and no other symptoms. His athletic trainer tells him to go home for the day and report back the next day. Over the course of the next several days, Connor's athletic trainer gradually increased the amount of physical activity he has him doing. He moves from stationary bicycling to jogging, from jogging to sprinting, and from sprinting to jumping, and cutting side to side. He then has Connor start cradling the lacrosse ball and passing with his teammates. He ultimately puts Connor in a practice with the rest of his teammates, but instructs him to step out during contact parts such as scrimmage, two-on-two drills, and gameplay. He even gives Connor a colored pinnie to remind him and all the others on the field that he is not to engage in contact drills. Connor is able to perform all these activities, including the sport-specific noncontact aspects of lacrosse, without any recurrence of his symptoms. Therefore, the athletic trainer repeats Connor's balance and neurocognitive assessments, noting that they are all comparable to his baseline performance prior to the start of the season when he was uninjured. Thus, the athletic trainer clears him to return to lacrosse. He is able to complete the remaining games of the season and ultimately finish the season without complication.

EXAMPLE 2: SPORT-RELATED CONCUSSION WITH PROLONGED RECOVERY

Rebecca is a 12-year-old soccer player in the sixth grade. She has been playing soccer for the last three years and has done so without any injuries, with the exception of a mild ankle sprain she suffered approximately two years ago. She is on offense as one of her teammates takes a corner kick.

As the ball is arcing toward Rebecca, she runs to meet it in an attempt to head it into the far corner of the goal. As she approaches the goal, however, the opposing goalie is also running full speed toward the ball. The goalie leaps into the air and extends her fists in an attempt to punch the ball out of the goal box. When she does so, one of her fist strikes Rebecca in the head. She falls to the ground where she remains for approximately 20 to 30 seconds. Her coach and her parents rush out to the field. It is clear that Rebecca is disoriented. She is uncertain as to who she is playing against, what time point in the game it is, and what the score is. She is complaining of a headache and feels sick to her stomach. Her parents take her to a local emergency department were she is examined. Fortunately, her examination is reassuring. The doctors tell Rebecca and her parents that she has suffered a sport-related concussion. They recommend that she avoid exercising and avoid performing tasks that require mental exertion such as reading, playing board games, card games, or video games, doing her homework, and other tasks that involve concentration and memory. Her parents take her home and she goes to bed relatively early that night. The remainder of the weekend, she lies on the couch and alternates between sleeping and simply listening to music. Her parents keep her home from school for several weeks, as she is still complaining of symptoms and they are following the instructions of the physician they saw in the emergency department. Two weeks after injury, her parents take Rebecca in to see her pediatrician to find out if there is anything else she should be doing. Rebecca's pediatrician confirms the diagnosis of concussion and recommends she continues to undergo physical and cognitive rest as instructed by the emergency department physician. As time goes on, Rebecca feels, if anything, worse than she did the first few days after injury. She is having difficulty falling asleep at night. Her headaches seem to be worse. She is becoming irritable and depressed. She misses her friends and is becoming worried that she is falling so far behind in school that she will be unable to make up the work and graduate on time with her friends going into the seventh grade next year. Furthermore, Rebecca feels dizzy when she tries to get up from the couch. She has low energy during the day and sleeps quite frequently. All in all, things do not appear to be going well. On a follow-up visit with her pediatrician roughly 5 weeks after injury, Rebecca and her parents report she seems to be getting worse. They are given a referral to a sports medicine specialist for her to see the following week. Given the duration of her symptoms and the fact that her symptoms are worsening, this physician orders several tests on Rebecca, including a picture of the brain known as an MRI. Fortunately, the MRI is normal. The brain is not bruised or bleeding, none of the cells are dying, there is no skull fracture, and there is no other abnormality that is causing Rebecca's symptoms. She is told by the sports medicine physician that indeed she does have a sport-related concussion. He offers her medicine that should reduce the intensity and frequency of her headaches. He recommends that she starts to gradually return to exercise beginning with stationary bicycling, with the goal of getting her back to exercising with the team while avoiding contact drills, and to ultimately return her to full soccer. He also recommends that she return to school and start making up the work she has missed. Rebecca and her parents are somewhat confused by the difference in recommendations between the sports medicine doctor, the doctors in the emergency room, and her pediatrician. Ultimately, however, they decide to start doing some light exercises and start returning her to school. Over the first few days back to school, Rebecca feels overwhelmed by the amount of work she has to do. She has difficulty following along in class. She develops worsening headaches and reports to the school nurse's office. On multiple occasions, she is sent home from school because of these headaches. Her symptoms continue to worsen, and ultimately they report back to her sports medicine physician. The doctor told her that this is to be expected, but not likely the result of her concussion. Rather, he suspects her current symptoms are due to the lack of exercise, missing soccer, and the circumstances of her being so far behind in school and the difficulties in catching up. He recommends that despite the symptoms, she remain in school and continue to make up work, continue to perform light aerobic exercise as was previously recommended. Gradually, as Rebecca does so over the next several weeks, her symptoms start to improve. She catches up in school and continues exercising. The exercise helps her fall asleep and stay asleep better during the evenings. Her headaches decrease, and the medicine seems to be effective. Dizziness is slowly resolving. In general, Rebecca is much happier. She is getting caught up in school, able to go to classes and see her friends, and able to see that someday she will be able to return to soccer.

Ultimately, three months after injury, Rebecca is symptom free. She is exercising with her team, including the skills training of soccer, but she is avoiding gameplay, two on two drills, and scrimmaging. Otherwise, she is sprinting and doing all forms of conditioning, dribbling the soccer ball, and she has remained symptom free. More importantly, she is completing her school work, including tests and quizzes. She is now taking a full course load and keeping up with her classmates. Her headache medication is discontinued and Rebecca remains symptom free.

The sports medicine physician has a long talk with Rebecca and her family now that she is symptom free, about when it is best to return her to soccer. Because she is so young, has a long soccer career ahead of her, had such a long recovery, and had such profound symptoms, the doctor recommends that Rebecca remain completely symptom free for several weeks before returning to contact sport. Furthermore, as Rebecca did not have any baseline data, the doctor reports that he believes she is completely recovered, but cannot say so for sure, as Rebecca did not have assessments of her balance or brain function at baseline, when uninjured, with which he can confirm she is completely recovered. Therefore, he recommends being more cautious in returning her to soccer. Ultimately, after this discussion, Rebecca and her family decide that, since she was not planning on participating in soccer during the summer and would not normally be participating until the autumn of the following year, she will spend the summer doing nonrisk noncontact drills of soccer and attending soccer skills camps. At the end of the summer, she will return to the sports medicine physician and have baseline measurements of her balance and brain function. Ultimately, she is able to return to play. She completes the following season injury free and symptom free.

EXAMPLE 3: MULTIPLE CONCUSSIONS, RISKS OUTWEIGH THE BENEFITS

Kenny is a fast runner. He has always been a fast runner. His freshman and sophomore year in high school he ran on the cross-country team and, although he was not the best on the team, he ran quite well and was a major contributor to the team and its overall success. He enjoyed it and it helped keep him in wonderful physical shape. Because of his success, speed, and athleticism, Kenny was approached by the high school football coach. The coach was interested in getting some more speed in the wide receiver and defensive back positions. He asked Kenny to consider coming out for the team. In addition, Kenny was approached by multiple classmates who played on the team. They were all very enthusiastic and supportive of the idea of Kenny participating in football his junior year. Also, Kenny was approached by several members of the cheerleading squad, including a girl he was quite fond of, who said they were looking forward to being able to cheer him on. After careful consideration, Kenny decided that he would like to play for the football team. He tried out and made the team. He played both offense and defense as a wide receiver and a defensive back. He also played on special teams.

Things seemed to be going quite well. Kenny was, as expected, a significant part of the team and was quite good at both his offensive and defensive position. It is in that setting, that on the fourth game of the season, Kenny received a kickoff and was running it back. He worked his way out to the 27-yard line when he was struck by one of his opponents.

It was a forceful blow, knocking Kenny backwards. When he landed, he struck the back of his head on the artificial turf quite forcefully. His helmet was knocked off his head. As Kenny attempted to rise to his feet, he fell to the ground. Ultimately, the team's athletic trainer and Kenny's coach came out on the field and he was removed from play. Since his examination and other tests did not reveal any other additional injuries, Kenny was diagnosed with a sport-related concussion and placed on physical and cognitive rest. His symptoms gradually improved over the following nine days. Ultimately, Kenny was symptom free. He was gradually returned to all cognitive and all nonrisk noncontact physical activities. He remained symptom free while he was sprinting, lifting weights, doing noncontact training drills, and performing all his schoolwork. He reported back to his athletic trainer, who repeated his baseline assessments in balance, cognition, and symptoms. He was noted to be back baseline in all measures and his athletic trainer was considering clearing Kenny to return to football. As he reviewed Kenny's medical file, however, he noticed that Kenny had previously sustained several other sport-related concussions. He was concerned given the number of concussions Kenny had sustained and worried he might be at risk for the cumulative effects of concussion. He had heard of some studies suggesting that perhaps American football players who sustained more than three concussions might be at increased risk for symptoms later in life. He therefore referred Kenny to a sports medicine physician in order to discuss this possibility further.

At the appointment with the sports medicine physician, Kenny was able to give the doctor great details about his concussions. Overall, during his lifetime, he had sustained three concussions. The first concussion he sustained was an accident that occurred when he slipped on some ice running to catch the school bus. He did not lose consciousness nor have amnesia with that injury. His symptoms lasted approximately four to five days after which time he was completely symptom free.

The second concussion occurred while he was participating in basketball; he was struck in the head by an elbow of one of his opponents. He had approximately one week of symptoms after that injury. He spent an additional week gradually returning to physical and cognitive activity. Ultimately, he was cleared to resume basketball and completed the season without additional injuries.

His third injury was the one he sustained during football.

Kenny, his parents, and the sports medicine physician had a long talk about the potential for cumulative effects of concussions sustained during sports. They discussed the risks of concussion in various sports, including American football, cross-country running, basketball, and other sports that Kenny was interested in. They discussed the literature describing the potential for risks later in life after multiple concussions, as well as the limitations of that literature. Ultimately, the doctor told Kenny he believed it would be safe for him to return to sports, including American football, which had the highest incidence of concussion among the sports Kenny was considering, if Kenny wished.

Kenny and his parents returned home and continued the discussion, weighing the risks of participating in football versus the benefits. There were clear benefits of participation in football. Kenny enjoyed the regular exercise associated with football. He enjoyed being part of the team and had made many new friends. As he was relatively good at football, playing gave him a certain amount of respect on campus, which had also resulted in him making many new friends. They also considered the risks involved. American football has a relatively high incidence of sport-related concussion as well as a relatively high incidence of other sport-related injuries. It was a fairly substantial time commitment that did detract, in part, from time he could spend on his other interests such as playing guitar and schoolwork. Kenny also noted that the risks of catastrophic injuries, such as cervical spinal injury and paralysis, were greater in American football than in cross-country running, basketball, or other sports he was interested in.

Ultimately, Kenny and his family decided that he could get similar benefits from participating in cross-country as he could from participating in American football. He was just as good at cross-country. Running cross country also gave him a certain amount of respect on campus. He enjoyed the exercise of running cross country, which also kept him in good physical shape. He had great friends on the cross-country team and his parents noted that running cross-country gave him equal benefits regarding his self-esteem. Furthermore, the risks involved in running cross-country were much lower than the risks of participating in American football, when it came to sport-related concussion and catastrophic injuries. Ultimately, Kenny and his family decided that the risks of participating in football outweighed the benefits and that the substantial benefits associated with participating in American football could be obtained from Kenny participating in cross-country. They therefore decided that he would no longer participate in American football, but rather, return to the cross-country team as his autumn sport. He would also continue participating in basketball during the winter and continue running track in the spring.

EXAMPLE 4: MULTIPLE CONCUSSIONS, BENEFITS OUTWEIGH THE RISKS

When he was a child, Bruce was really not very physically active. He enjoyed playing video games and watching television, after he was finished doing his homework. He grew up in a rather rough section of town and his mother did not let him go outside to play at the playground where there was often violent episodes, including gunfire. She was worried that he might get injured or get into trouble with the local gangs that hung out there. Therefore, Bruce spent most of this time in their small apartment building. He was, however, relatively athletic. Bruce was big for his age, always standing a few inches taller than most of his classmates. He was overweight for sure, but he was always picked early on when his classmates were picking teams during recess or gym class. Still, he was self-conscious about his looks and physicality, as he was always overweight compared to most of his classmates. His mother felt that, in part, this resulted in his having low self-esteem, a poor image of himself, and a lack of confidence. He would get picked on at school fairly frequently. His grades were, for the most part, below average. His mother was concerned that this was due to the difficult time he was having at school, constantly being teased by other children.

When he started the seventh grade, however, may of his classmates told him that given his size he might be good at playing football. The team was short of linemen that year, and they thought that given his abilities demonstrated during gym class, he could be a big, strong, lineman in football and could add to the team. Bruce tried out for the team and ended up being one of the better players. He really enjoyed playing football, as he became friends with all the other boys on the team. He was so good at football, the kids in his class stopped picking on him. Even his mother could see his own self-image improve dramatically. He became quite confident. He looked forward to going to school every day. He had friends coming over to his house regularly. His grades began to improve. And his mother noticed that he became physically more fit. He was still overweight, but he became more muscular, stood more upright, and the relative proportion of his belly in relation to his muscles seemed to decrease. Overall, Bruce was growing into a strong, confident, proud young man.

At the end of seventh grade football, Bruce tried out for the basketball team. Although he was not as good at basketball as he was at football, many of the players on the football team also played basketball. Bruce enjoyed being with them an additional season, maintaining their friendships throughout the winter. He threw the shot put and discus with the track team during the spring. Overall, Bruce really became a much greater member of the student body. His grades continued to improve over the course of the year, as did his physique. So inspired by his abilities in sports, his new-found friendships, and the improvement in his grades, Bruce decided that, over the summer, he would continue training. He started a regimen of aerobic activity, including jogging, stationary bicycling, and working out on the rowing machine. He continued resistance training, working with the athletic trainer at school to come up with a regimen of weightlifting exercises to improve his strength. When he returned to school in the eighth grade, he again joined the junior high football team. He became best friends with the quarterback, who was one of the more popular kids in school. His grades continued to improve as did his overall physicality. He went in for his annual physical at the pediatrician's office and the pediatrician noted that the measurements of his body fat and body mass index had improved substantially over the course of the previous year. He talked with Bruce about how the other measures of his health seemed to be improving as well. The pediatrician recommended that Bruce continue participating in sports.

Unfortunately, in November, Bruce was on defense and went to tackle a running back on the opposing team, when he was simultaneously struck in the head by an opposing blocker, knocking him to the ground. He developed headaches and dizziness. Bruce reported to his athletic trainer who diagnosed him with a sport-related concussion and placed him on relative physical and cognitive rest. After the symptoms resolved, in a matter of 11 days, the athletic trainer began returning Bruce to exercise and to full academic activity accordingly. He remained completely symptom free for a total of two weeks, when his athletic trainer repeated all his baseline assessments and noted that they were all comparable to his pre-injury baseline scores in every assessment. The athletic trainer was considering clearing him for sports and instructed Bruce to follow-up with his pediatrician. During that visit, it was noted that Bruce had sustained two previous sport-related concussions during gym class in grade school. One was sustained during dodge ball when he was struck in the face by a ball thrown forcefully by one of his classmates. He had approximately three days' worth of symptoms with that injury. The second concussion occurred when he fell while playing floor hockey during gym class and he struck his head on the floor. He had approximately nine days of symptoms with that injury.

The pediatrician discussed with Bruce and his mother the potential for cumulative effects of concussions that occur during sports. He discussed with them the medical and scientific evidence suggesting the cumulative effects of concussion as well as the limitations of those studies. He asked Bruce and his mother to weigh the risks and benefits of continuing to participate in sports, particularly American football, and come back the following week to continue the discussion.

Over the course of that week, Bruce and his mother involved his coaches, his older brother who also was a football player, and several other people important in their lives in the discussion. All had noticed that Bruce was deriving many great benefits from his participation in football. For the first time in his life, he was getting regular exercise; he enjoyed the exercise. He made more friends at school. His own self-image and self-esteem improved markedly. His grades improved markedly, as had his overall health. And, most importantly, Bruce really enjoyed playing American football. Even the brief length of time that he had been in active recovery, his mother had noticed that he seemed more depressed and withdrawn, as if he was perhaps losing confidence and looking more like his former self.

They also understood the risks involved in participating in American football. The incidence of sport-related concussion was higher in American football than most other high school team sports. They also knew the risk of catastrophic injury was somewhat high, as were the risks of other injuries such as fractures, ligament sprains, and muscle and tendon strains. After carefully considering these risks against the benefits Bruce derived from participation in football, he and his mother decided that the benefits far outweighed the risks. His participation in football had changed Bruce's life. For the first time, he was considering attending college. He was actively interested in his grades. He exhibited greater self-confidence, enjoyment of school, enjoyment of social relationships. They therefore made the decision to return him to football. They discussed their thoughts with his pediatrician and he was given a letter clearing him medically to return to football. He participated in the remainder of the season, including the state championship. Unfortunately, his team lost the state championship. Nonetheless, he was delighted to be part of the team and delighted to be able to compete in the game.

SUMMARY

In summary, the recovery from sport-related concussion varies among athletes. While most high school athletes will recover quite quickly, some will have longer recoveries. In addition, athletes who sustain multiple injuries have severe difficulties after injury, have profound symptoms after injury, or other complicating factors will be managed differently than those with straightforward recoveries. When deciding whether or not to return athletes who recover from sport-related concussions to their chosen sports, the athletes, the athletes' parents, and all treating physicians must weigh the benefits to that particular athlete obtained from returning to their chosen sports against the risks involved in participating in their chosen sports. After carefully considering these risks and benefits, they must come to a conclusion as to whether or not the benefits outweigh the risks. If so, the athlete will return to sport. Alternatively, if the risks outweigh the benefits, athletes must make the difficult decision to not return to their sports.

CHAPTER 11

Medical Research and the Future of Sport-Related Concussion

It is always difficult to predict what the future holds. This is particularly true in the realm of medicine and science, where new discoveries are made every day and new developments are published daily. There is so much effort being put in to discovering better ways to diagnose, quantify, treat, and prevent sport-related concussions it is hard to keep up with it all, even for those of us who spend the majority of our time on this particular issue. Still, being able to see and read about the work that is currently underway, it is reasonable to try and guess what things will be useful in the future.

PREDICTORS OF INJURY

It is possible that certain athletes are more susceptible to sustaining sport-related concussions than others. One can imagine that certain predisposing factors may increase the risk for certain athletes. Given the relationship between the neck muscles and the resultant spinning of the brain after a collision, it is possible that athletes who have neck muscles of a certain size, shape, strength, length, or other factors may be at different risk for sport-related concussion. While some of these, such as neck muscle strength, are modifiable in that the athlete can increase his or her neck muscle strength, others, such as the shape, location of the attachments of the muscles to the underlying bones, and length of the muscles, are not readily modifiable. They may be used, however, to predict who is at high risk for sport-related concussion. For example, if studies revealed that an athlete whose neck muscles were longer were at increased risk for sport-related concussion, then we could, in theory, measure neck muscle length and use it as a way of quantifying the risk of injury, helping to gauge the risk of concussion. This information might guide the athlete when making decisions regarding which sports to participate in or whether not to return to certain sports after having sustained a sport-related concussion.

Similarly, there may be a genetic predisposition to concussion for some. Certain genes have already been explored as possibly being related to the risk of sport-related concussion or to the risk of developing prolonged recovery or long-term problems as a result of sport-related concussions. One commonly discussed gene in this area is the gene apolipoprotein E epsilon 4, or APOE 4 for short. As of yet, the evidence regarding APOE 4 and its relation to sport-related concussion or possible consequences after sport-related concussions is too preliminary to make it a useful tool. That, however, is not to say that it will not be useful in predicting injury or outcomes after injury in the future. Furthermore, it is only one of thousands of genes, any of which may be related to the incidence of sport-related concussion or the potential for long-term problems resulting from multiple sport-related concussions. It would not be surprising if, sometime over the next few years, researchers discovered a gene or perhaps several genes that are related to either the risk of suffering sport-related concussions or the risk of developing long-term problems from concussions sustained during sports.

BIOMARKERS

Another developing area of concussion involves what are known as biomarkers. Throughout the text, it has hopefully become apparent that we do not yet have a way of definitively diagnosing concussion or determining when an athlete has completely recovered from a concussion. Biomarkers are measurements that might be taken from the athletes that would do precisely this—allow us to definitively diagnose whether or not an athlete has sustained a concussion and allow us to definitively determine when an athlete has recovered from a concussion. Already, several biomarkers have been proposed and tested. Many of these are the measurements of products in the blood. Some commonly discussed ones are known as glial fibrillary acidic protein (GFAP), S100 B, and neuron specific enolase (NSE), among others. In addition, the deposition of abnormal form of the protein hyperphosphorylated cis tau, discussed earlier, in the chapter on chronic traumatic encephalopathy, has been measured in athletes in various ways after sporting events. That is to say, when athletes are young and unlikely to have developed CTE, but have sustained blows to the head and/or concussions during recent athletic activity, one might measure the amount of hyper-phosphorylated cis tau in their blood or saliva. This might be used to help diagnose or determine recovery from a sport-related concussion, or might be useful as a means of predicting whether or not an athlete is susceptible to suffering long-term consequences from concussions sustained during sports. There are many other biomarkers currently under investigation. Although the data are too preliminary to definitively say one way or another which, if any, will be useful in the future, they are promising.

Currently, while images of the brain in the form of magnetic resonance imaging (MRI) and computed tomography (CT) are useful in diagnosing skull fractures, blood in the brain, swelling in the brain, and other injuries and abnormalities of the brain, they are not yet capable of diagnosing a concussion or determining recovery from a concussion. Furthermore, these images do not yet allow us to determine whether or not former athletes have developed chronic traumatic encephalopathy. Studies are actively being undertaken, however, at prestigious medical schools in the country to try and determine whether or not an athlete has a concussion or is still in active recovery from a concussion. Similarly, studies are underway to try and determine whether or not athletes who sustained concussions in sports and are now older have developed chronic traumatic encephalopathy. This includes imaging modalities being investigated to determine whether or not the presence and distribution of abnormal hyperphosphorylated cis tau can be detected in athletes while they are still alive.

TREATMENTS

Finally, there are treatments for concussion as well as possible the long-term effects of concussion currently being studied. Some of the more promising involve physical therapy, vestibular therapy, and ocular therapy. As noted earlier, concussion can result in difficulties with balance, coordination, and vision. Furthermore, because athletes are restricted from exercising shortly after their concussion, and regular exercise is associated with the regulation of blood flow to the brain, lack of exercise can lead to a disturbance in the way that blood flow to the brain is regulated. Physical therapists, and subspecialists within the field of physical therapy known as vestibular therapists, can guide athletes through a series of exercises that may reduce these symptoms, particularly those related to dizziness, vision, poor coordination. Furthermore, by safely guiding athletes through a gradual return to exercise, some of the symptoms that are due to restrictions in exercise may also resolve.

Other therapies may also be developed that will help the underlying cellular problem that results in the symptoms of concussion. One therapy which has been studied in animals as well as people who develop chronic symptoms from concussion involves the transmission of light in a certain color spectrum, a certain wavelength, to the cells of the brain by shining through the skin and scalp. This treatment, which has become known as light-emitting diode therapy, is still under investigation. It is unclear yet whether or not it will help those recovering from brain injury, but has shown some promise.

There may also be medications that could be useful in the treatment of concussion. Right now, medications are used for alleviating some of the symptoms that occur after sport-related concussions. There may be, in the future, a medication that is useful for correcting the underlying problem with the cells.

Furthermore, treatments designed to decrease the risk of long-term problems from concussion including chronic traumatic encephalopathy may be developed in the future. Some of these therapies may be quite simple and easy to implement. For example, it has been shown that by separating concussions over time, allowing for greater amount of time to pass prior to additional injury, the potential for long-term problems with memory and the ability to learn in animals has decreased. If the same holds true for athletes, one would need only increase the period of rest athletes must undergo in between recovering from a concussion and being allowed to return to play, in order to decrease their risk of developing problems with memory and learning in the future. It may also affect the risk of other symptoms in the future such as headaches and other symptoms that we are unable to study effectively in animals.

Furthermore, animal models of concussion and repeated concussion have resulted in the accumulation of hyperphosphorylated cis tau in the brains of these animals. An antibody has been developed which, in animal studies, has been shown to block the progression of hyperphosphorylated cis tau after injury. If it turns out that hyperphosphorylated cis tau is, in fact, the underlying problem that causes the symptoms experienced by former athletes later in life, then blocking hyperphosphorylated cis tau with this antibody and preventing its spread could potentially decrease the risk of those symptoms, decrease the risk of what is known today as chronic traumatic encephalopathy.

SUMMARY

In summary, it is always difficult to predict the future, particularly in medicine and science. There does, however, appear to be promising developments that in the future may allow us to predict who is at highest risk of sustaining sport-related concussions or who is at highest risk for suffering long-term consequences of repeated sport-related concussions. There may be ways of measuring, definitively diagnosing, and definitively determining recovery from concussions known as biomarkers. We may develop imaging techniques that will help diagnose concussion, determine recovery from concussion, diagnose chronic traumatic encephalopathy, or other long-term consequences that result from repeated sport-related concussions. There may also be therapy that will directly treat the underlying processes that result in concussion or perhaps treat or prevent the development of long-term consequences of repeated concussion, up to and including chronic traumatic encephalopathy.

CHAPTER 12

Epidemiology: The Study of the Frequency and Determinants of Disease

Epidemiology is the study of the frequency, distribution, and determinants of disease or injury. While a thorough review of epidemiology is beyond the scope of this text and not required for understanding the controversies involved in the area of concussion, we will need to understand some of the basic principles of epidemiology in order to understand the controversy surrounding concussion and sport-related concussion in particular. These controversies can only be well-understood if the reader understands how the studies of concussion, its frequency in sports, and the determinants of injury, recovery, and cumulative effects were conducted. Therefore, this chapter will give a brief review of the scientific method and discuss some fundamental principles of epidemiology that will later be used to further our discussion of the controversies.

It may come as a shock to some readers to learn that there is no single study that proves that smoking cigarettes causes lung cancer. To be sure, smoking cigarettes does cause lung cancer. There is no longer any question about that. However, the reason we know that smoking is associated with an increased risk of lung cancer stems from a series of epidemiological studies, none of which, in isolation, proves that smoking causes lung cancer. But, when taken together, the overall body of evidence clearly demonstrates that smoking leads to lung cancer. Following this example through will help us understand better how medical research is conducted and how we learn which factors are associated with an increased risk of disease. In doing so, we will then be able to apply what we have learned to the topic of concussions and better understand the controversies involved.

Prior to discussing epidemiology, let us first discuss the scientific method. For most readers, this will be a review of something they have learned in their basic science classes in grammar school, junior high school, and certainly by the time of high school. The scientific method is a process for experimenting that is used in most fields of science. It is used to explore observations, develop hypotheses that explain those observations, and test the hypotheses in order to ultimately develop a theory. We use it to determine the cause and effect relationships that occur in nature as well as in medicine. Reviewing the scientific process helps us to better understand epidemiology and the controversies involved in the study of concussion. The scientific method dictates that in the quest to discover the truth, an investigator must start by making an observation. To continue with our example of smoking tobacco and the risk of lung cancer, some physicians and scientists, way back when, noted that lung cancer seems to be fairly common among people who smoke tobacco products. For reasons we will learn shortly, this observation alone is not sufficient evidence that smoking tobacco products causes lung cancer.

It could be that people who smoke tobacco products engage in other behaviors more commonly than people who do not smoke, and that it is these other behaviors that lead to the increased risk of lung cancer. It could be that smoking is more common among those people that carry a certain gene, and that this gene is associated with an increased risk of lung cancer. It could be that smokers are more likely to develop a cough that leads to a doctor ordering an X-ray. Therefore, even if the risk of lung cancer were the same between smokers and nonsmokers, smokers would be more likely to be diagnosed, as they would be more likely to have an X-ray that reveals the cancer than nonsmokers. Thus, doctors would think smokers were more likely to have lung cancer, but really, they are just more likely to have their cancer discovered, because they are more likely to get an X-ray.

Still, making an observation, while insufficient by itself to prove an association between a risk factor and a disease, is the necessary initial step in the scientific method. It is only once the observation is made that investigators can proceed to the second step of the scientific method—developing an hypothesis that is based on the observation. One logical hypothesis in our example would be that smoking tobacco products causes lung cancer or increases the risk of lung cancer. Still, as discussed above, this hypothesis may not be accurate. Therefore, once this hypothesis has been developed, it must be tested. Testing of the hypothesis is the third step of the scientific method. This is where epidemiology comes in. Epidemiology is used to test hypotheses that were developed and based on observations. The different methods for testing of hypotheses will be discussed later in this chapter. Once the hypothesis has been tested using various methods, the findings from all the different studies used to test the hypothesis are considered, and a conclusion is reached. If they are all pointing in the same direction—in other words, all indicating that smoking tobacco products increases the risk of developing lung cancer—then the investigators conclude that smoking is associated with an increased risk of lung cancer. This process of reaching a conclusion represents the fourth step of the scientific method. In a more simply stated form, the steps of the scientific method are:

1. Make an observation.
2. Develop an hypothesis that explains the observation.
3. Test that hypothesis in multiple different ways, in varying situations, with varying approaches.
4. Reach a conclusion based on the findings of the tests conducted in Step 3.

Many of the studies used in medicine parallel the scientific method. The simplest form of medical study consists of merely reporting observations. New, novel, interesting, or unusual observations are reported in what is known as a case report. Sticking with our original example, prior to the common knowledge about tobacco smoke and lung cancer, one physician may have observed that one of his patients who developed lung cancer was a particularly heavy smoker. In other words, this patient may have smoked an unusually large number of cigarettes per day, and may have done so for many years. Making that observation, he may have written up the case in a medical journal article, describing the amount of cigarettes per day that this patient smoked, the number of years that this patient had been smoking such a large number of cigarettes, and the medical symptoms that the patient developed leading ultimately to the diagnosis of a lung cancer. If such a case study were reported, the physician may have hypothesized that perhaps the frequent use of cigarettes by this patient was associated with the development of lung cancer.

A stronger, albeit still highly limited, method of reporting such an observation is what is known as a case series. In a case series, the physician would not have noticed a single patient who developed lung cancer after a long history of smoking, but rather noticed that in his or her practice there were several patients who developed lung cancer, all of them particularly heavy cigarette smokers, consuming a large number of cigarettes per day for many years. This would be a series of observations as opposed to just one observation. As above, the physician would describe in what is known as case series, the amount of cigarettes per day that each of these patients smoked, the number of years during which each had been smoking such a large number of cigarettes, and the medical symptoms that each patient experienced that ultimately led to the diagnosis of lung cancer. While a case series is somewhat stronger than a simple case report, it is still limited in its ability to allow the scientist to draw conclusions. Rather, case series are used, much like case reports, to generate an hypothesis. In our example, the hypothesis would be similar to the one developed from the case report: smoking tobacco products is associated with an increased risk of lung cancer.

Once developed, researchers then need to test the hypothesis. There are several ways of doing so. One way is conducting what is called a case-control study. In a case-control study, we start with a sample population consisting of some members who have a particular disease and those that do not. In other words, the outcome you are interested in has already occurred. To continue with our current example, we would find a population of people, say in your local geographic area or town, and separate them into two groups: those who have lung cancer and those who do not. The participants with lung cancer would be considered the cases and those without lung cancer would be the controls. We would then try to determine the level of exposure to various risk factors that we hypothesize are associated with the outcome, and see if the level of exposure to each differs between the cases and controls. Continuing with our current example, we would ask both members with lung cancer and those without to try and recall how many cigarettes they smoked per day, on average, over the course of how many years. We would also assess other risk factors that we hypothesized were associated with lung cancer, such as high-fat diets. Therefore, we would ask them what their typical daily diet was like. We might also ask how frequently they engaged in aerobic exercise, how much alcohol they drank per week, and whether or not they had other health problems. We might ask where they were employed, as we might hypothesize that people who worked in asbestos factories, in coal mines, or in other conditions where they breathe in a lot of dirty air were also at increased risk for lung cancer. By doing so, we might notice that those participants who had lung cancer smoked more tobacco over a longer period of time than those participants who did not have lung cancer. Such a finding would strengthen our hypothesis that smoking is associated with an increased risk of lung cancer.

Another method for studying disease and risk factors is known as a cohort study. A cohort is defined as a population or group of people who are observed by investigators over time. Cohorts, representing people in a certain geographic area or town, are then followed and every year or so investigators will ask the members of cohorts to give them some information about their daily living habits, whether or not they smoke tobacco products and if so how often, whether or not they drink alcohol and if so how much, how frequently they exercise, what their diet consists of, what their occupation is, health problems suffered by them and their immediate genetic family members, and other similar parameters. As with any population, over time, some of these individuals will become sick while most will remain healthy. Again, continuing with our current example, the goal is to determine risk factors for lung cancer. As members of the cohort develop lung cancer, the investigators will go back to the information they collected and try to determine the difference between those members that went on to develop lung cancer and those that did not. If such investigators observe that members of the cohort that were smoking tobacco products were more likely to develop lung cancer, then this would further strengthen the hypothesis that smoking is related to the risk of lung cancer. Note that one key difference between case-control studies and cohort studies is that, in a case-control study, the outcome has already occurred—some members of the study had already developed lung cancer. In a cohort study, however, the population is healthy at the start. Data are collected before the outcome has occurred, before any of the participants have lung cancer.

The final method of study that we will be discussing in brief is called a randomized controlled trial. In a randomized controlled trial, the investigator hypothesizes that certain risk factors are associated with an increased risk of a given disease. The investigator then randomly assigns some participants to be exposed to that risk factor while preventing others from being exposed. As the study continues, the investigators observe which group is most likely to develop the disease; do, in fact, the members exposed to the risk factor have a higher occurrence of the disease than those not exposed? If we were to do this using our current example, we would take a group of people and randomly assigned some of them to start smoking cigarettes. We would instruct the others to never smoke cigarettes. As time went on, we would see whether or not the ones who smoked cigarettes were at increased risk of developing lung cancer. Obviously, conducting such an experiment would be unethical, as we know that smoking increases the risk of many health-related problems, including lung cancer. This type of study would never be conducted. There are, however, situations where these studies are conducted, particularly when the population stands to derive a benefit from the results. Just to illustrate, we might hypothesize that men over certain age who take a low dose of aspirin every day are less likely to suffer heart attacks. In order to answer test this hypothesis, we might take a group of men and give some of them a low dose of aspirin every day. We might instruct others not to take aspirin. Over the following years, we would then observe whether the men taking aspirin were less likely to have heart attacks than those not taking aspirin. Since the risks of taking daily a low dose of aspirin are low, there is little risk to those in the group recommended to that regimen. Since you are conducting the study, the benefits of taking a daily low dose of aspirin must be unknown, and therefore, there is little risk to the group who is instructed *not* to take daily aspirin. Thus, this example is much more probable than the one above, where certain participants are instructed to smoke cigarettes.

All these different types of studies have certain advantages and disadvantages. While we will not review all the advantages and disadvantages involved in each of these study designs, there are a few that will be relevant to our discussion of controversies within the area of concussion, and therefore we will discuss them in detail now.

In a case report or case series, an investigator reports an observation. In our example, patients who develop lung cancer appear to be heavy smokers. Case reports and case series are excellent ways to generate an hypothesis. They do not, however, represent evidence by themselves. The observation may be incorrect, misleading, incomplete, or otherwise inaccurate. The observations described by case series or case reports need to lead to further investigations, tests of the hypotheses they generate, in order to reach the ultimate goal of guiding us to the truth. Nonetheless, there can be no hypotheses to test without first making an observation. This is why it is the first step of the scientific method and why case reports along with case series are essential to the scientific process.

A specific limitation of case-control studies is known as recall bias. As discussed above, in case-control studies the outcome of interest, in our example lung cancer, has already occurred. Some members of the study have lung cancer while other members do not. We, then, ask participants to give us information about potential risk factors to which they were exposed over time. In essence, we ask participants to recall, previously, over the course of their life, how many cigarettes they smoked, how many alcohol-containing beverages they drank, how much fat their diet contained, how often they exercised, how many hours a week they slept, and other such factors. Recall bias is a commonly discussed phenomenon in epidemiology where subjects inaccurately recall their exposures to various risk factors, based on whether or not they have the disease in question.

More simply put, people who know they have a disease may recall their exposure to various risk factors differently than those without disease. Given the public attention paid to various risk factors, environmental exposures, and personal habits, many people already have in their minds ideas as to whether or not certain exposures are good for them. It is, therefore, possible that those who suffer from a certain disease may recall more accurately or even overestimate their exposure to given risk factors than those without. In our example, those that know they have lung cancer may be able to recall with vivid memory the amount of cigarettes they had over the course of their lifetime. They may even overestimate the amount they smoked as they now know they have lung cancer and, therefore, assume they must have had a fairly high exposure to tobacco smoke. A similar person who does not have lung cancer may not recall or may underestimate the amount of exposure he or she had previously to cigarette smoke. This phenomenon is known as recall bias.

Another limitation in medical research is known as confounding. Confounding leads an investigator to consider one factor to be associated with a disease, when in reality a different, unmeasured factor is the culprit. Confounding occurs when a given exposure is associated with an outcome as well as another potential risk factor. A confounding variable is one that is associated with a given risk factor and with the occurrence of the disease. If investigators are focusing on one risk factor, but do not consider a potential confounding variable, they may inaccurately determine that the original risk factor is associated with disease when, in fact, it is not. Although this is complicated to read about in general terms, using our example may help illustrate this phenomenon more clearly.

If investigators are trying to determine the risk factors for developing lung cancer by collecting information on a large number of participants, they may notice that participants who drink large amounts of alcohol are more likely to develop lung cancer. Therefore, they may conclude that drinking alcohol increases the risk of developing lung cancer. It could be, however, that people who drink large quantities of alcohol are more likely to smoke cigarettes than those who drink less or do not drink at all. While it is the smoking that leads to an increased risk of lung cancer, if the investigators neither considered nor measured cigarette smoking as a risk factor, they would have observed that those drinking large amounts of alcohol had higher rates of lung cancer. Therefore, they may have concluded that alcohol was associated with an increased risk of developing lung cancer. In this scenario, cigarette smoking is a confounding variable, one that is associated with both the variable of interest, alcohol intake, and the outcome, lung cancer.

Summary

In summary, the scientific method demands that an investigator first make an observation. In the medical literature, observations are often reported as case reports or case series. Investigators then develop an hypothesis based on those observations. The hypothesis is then tested in various ways, some of which are case-control studies, cohort studies, and randomized control trials. If the testing of an hypothesis in multiple different ways leads to the same conclusions, say that the heavy smoking of cigarettes is associated with an increased risk of lung cancer, then the investigators draw a conclusion: smoking causes lung cancer. All forms of study have limitations. One limitation, known as recall bias, occurs when participants with a known disease or injury are more likely to recall exposure to given risk factor than participants without the disease or injury. Another limitation, known as confounding, occurs when one risk factor appears associated with disease, but in reality is associated with a different risk factor that is associated with the disease, thereby misleading the investigator.

SECTION II

Controversies

CHAPTER 13

Issues Surrounding Definition and Diagnosis

As described earlier, concussion is a disturbance of brain function that occurs due to rotational acceleration. It is a traumatic brain injury. The diagnosis of concussion is made by taking a medical history and performing a physical examination. There are currently no tests that are able to "see" or otherwise definitively measure a concussion. Classically, an athlete reports experiencing some trauma to the head, followed by typical symptoms of concussion such as headaches, difficulty with concentration, nausea, and other similar symptoms. Based on this history, a diagnosis of concussion is made. These symptoms, however, are nonspecific. That is to say, they are not only the symptoms of concussion, but also other medical conditions or injuries. For example, dehydration, which occurs commonly during sports, can result in headaches, dizziness, difficulty concentrating, drowsiness, a feeling of being "out of it," and several other symptoms that are also associated with concussion. Similarly, depression, viral illness, emotional stress, lack of sleep, caffeine withdrawal, and many other entities may also result in the symptoms associated with concussion. Therefore, a history of trauma to the head that resulted in the symptoms is crucial when making the diagnosis of concussion.

Given the increased scrutiny of over the management of concussions occurring during sports, there is now a heightened sensitivity among athletes, coaches, athletic trainers, and sports medicine physicians to diagnose concussions. This has led to many diagnoses of concussion among athletes that are experiencing any of these symptoms, and also participating in a sport where concussions are common, such as American football, ice hockey, soccer, basketball, lacrosse, and others. Often, athletes will come to the clinic complaining of a headache and not feeling quite right. They do not recall any incident where they were struck in the head or experienced some other rapid rotational acceleration of their head, and yet, they are concerned they have a concussion. Many times, these athletes will be formally diagnosed with a concussion by their medical provider, even in the absence of any identifiable trauma, simply because they are experiencing these symptoms and they participate in a sport in which concussions are fairly common. Some argue that, given the risks involved with returning an athlete to play prior to full recovery from a concussion, it is better to err on the side of caution—remove these athletes from play and treat them as if they have suffered a concussion so that they are not placed at an increased risk of further blows to the head, second impact syndrome, worsening of symptoms, or an elongated recovery.

Others, however, have argued that these symptoms are so nonspecific and so common that many athletes experiencing these symptoms would be misdiagnosed with concussion leading to several possible harms. First, once they are diagnosed with a concussion and managed accordingly, they and their medical providers would likely stop searching for other potential causes; the real cause of their symptoms might go undetected and untreated, thereby prolonging their recovery. Second, athletes with a concussion are restricted from their activities, including sports. These restrictions are associated with symptoms of their own, including many associated with concussions such as sleep disturbance, headaches, dizziness, depression, fatigue, and irritability, among others. Thus, diagnosing these athletes erroneously with a concussion might prolong and even exacerbate their symptoms. This might lead to further restrictions on their activities, thereby worsening their condition. Third, as athletes accumulate sport-related concussions, they increase their risk of potential cumulative effects of concussions. Thus, many athletes, parents, coaches, and sports medicine providers keep track of the number of concussions an athlete has sustained, and use that number as one factor when making decisions about whether or not an athlete should return to his or her sport. An erroneous diagnosis of concussion adds an extra concussion to the overall total number and may lead to the unnecessary, premature removal from sports. And, while preventing the potential cumulative effects from concussions is important, today's children are at far greater risk of the potential effects of inactivity, such as obesity, diabetes, heart disease, stroke, mood disorders, low self-esteem, and many other conditions, which can be prevented by the regular exercise associated with sports participation, than they are of the potential cumulative effects from concussions. Finally, if athletes grow concerned that when they mention symptoms to their medical care providers they will be diagnosed with a concussion, even in the absence of head trauma, they may be reluctant to report their symptoms, thus leading to undiagnosed and improperly managed concussions.

Given the inability for doctors and scientists to "see" a concussion on modern-day imaging such as computed tomography (CT) or magnetic resonance imaging (MRI), or to diagnose concussion through a blood test, or to otherwise definitively measure a concussion, there is current controversy about how the diagnosis should be made. Dehydration occurs commonly during sports, particularly during the hot temperatures of summer and early fall. One can imagine that the dehydrated athlete with the common symptoms of dehydration, headaches, dizziness, fatigue, might have experienced a blow or even several blows to the head over the course of a game. In this setting, it can be difficult to distinguish the symptoms of dehydration from those of a concussion. If the athlete is completely symptom free, but sustains a blow to the head followed immediately by the symptoms, then concussion becomes the most likely diagnosis. In the absence of one clear blow triggering symptoms, dehydration becomes the more likely diagnosis. But without a definitive test or measure of concussion, the diagnosis is unclear.

This type of situation has led to controversy about how the diagnosis of concussion should be made. Many argue that, given the risks of returning athletes to their sports while they are still incompletely recovered from their concussion, we should be conservative and make the diagnosis anytime an athlete is experiencing signs or symptoms that can be caused by concussion. Others have argued that because the signs and symptoms of concussion are nonspecific and can be caused by other injuries and medical conditions, the diagnosis should be made more cautiously. Specifically, they argue there should be an obvious history of trauma and ideally some other objective measurement of concussion such as a disturbance in balance or a decrease in neurocognitive performance.

There is a concern that athletes, in particular, who are at increased risk for concussion, may develop the symptoms often associated with concussions due to other reasons. For example, one can imagine that the student–athlete, who is applying to colleges and is under enormous amount of pressure to succeed, might develop symptoms related to the emotional stress of the college application process. It is not uncommon for there to be substantial anxiety around academic performance, particularly during the last two to three years of high school. This anxiety and emotional stress often results in difficulty falling asleep or remaining asleep. Such disturbance in sleep may lead to headaches, difficulty concentrating, fatigue, depression, the feeling of being out of it, drowsiness, and many other symptoms that can also occur with concussion. If athletes experiencing these symptoms happen to play a sport in which the risk of concussion is substantial, they may be misdiagnosed with a concussion. If this were the case, the true cause of their symptoms— anxiety and emotional stress— may remain untreated. Therefore, their symptoms would likely progress under the mistaken belief that they were due to a concussion.

Others worry that perhaps student athletes might have an incentive to report being concussed and report prolonged symptoms of concussion. As noted earlier, one of the treatments for concussion involves cognitive rest. As student athletes undergo cognitive rest, doctors will often reduce their workload so that they are taking fewer courses than they otherwise would. Furthermore, some may be given academic accommodations, which allow them to decrease the amount of work they have to do and increase the amount of time they have to do their remaining schoolwork. Some fear that athletes may, therefore, report concussions and persistent symptoms of concussion in order to have these academic accommodations. This is one of the reasons why schools will often require an athlete make up any missed work, once they are recovered from a concussion, to counteract this type of incentive. It is important that they learn that material before they progress to the next grade. But it is also a deterrent to embellishing symptoms of concussion.

Still, others believe that the current criteria for diagnosing a concussion are not stringent enough. As discussed previously, there is currently no medical test that can be done to confirm the diagnosis of concussion. Doctors, athletic trainers, and other medical care providers are highly reliant on a history that is reported to them for the patient; if patients do not report their symptoms, most concussion will go undiagnosed. As it has been well studied and shown that athletes often neglect to report the symptoms of a concussion, relying on them to report their symptoms likely results in many concussion going undiagnosed.

The timing of concussion symptoms is also a source of controversy and debate. As mentioned previously, the signs and symptoms of concussion start at the time of impact or shortly thereafter. There have been, however, reports of athletes who were diagnosed with a concussion because three or four days after a blow to the head they began experiencing symptoms such as headaches, dizziness, and other symptoms often associated with concussion. As there is no definitive test with which the diagnosis of concussion can be confirmed, however, it is unclear whether or not these athletes have sustained concussions with a delayed onset of symptoms or whether their symptoms are due to something unrelated to the blow to the head and are, therefore, not due to a concussion at all. This is a common occurrence in sports. Clearly, symptoms that begin at the moment of impact and are gradually resolving are likely to be due to a concussion, and symptoms that begin several weeks after a blow to the head are unlikely to be due to concussion. It is not uncommon, however, for athletes to report a blow to the head that was followed by symptoms that are associated with concussion that started several hours or a few days after the blow to the head. In these situations, it is unclear what the cause of the symptoms is. Some experts argue that they should be diagnosed with a concussion and that the delayed onset of symptoms is a rare but actual occurrence. Others argue that the signs and symptoms of concussion, particularly given the current hypothesis regarding the pathophysiology of concussion, begin immediately and that the delayed onset of symptoms are not in fact symptoms of concussion but rather symptoms of some other process.

This particular controversy is exacerbated by our current understanding of what a concussion is, what happens to the brain when it suffers a concussion, the pathophysiology of concussion.

Please recall that in Chapter 2 we discussed the physiology and pathophysiology of concussion. That is to say, we learned how the cells of the brain operated normally by conducting action potentials, and how concussion caused the disruption of their ability to send these action potentials by deforming the cell membrane and allowing large amounts of sodium ions to move from the outer, extracellular space, through sodium-potassium channels and into the cell. We further learned that in order to pump the sodium back outside the cell, the neurons require ATP. ATP is delivered to the brain ultimately from the bloodstream; there is decreased blood flow to the brain after concussion. This mismatch between an increased demand for ATP and a decreased delivery of ATP results in the signs and symptoms of concussion. This hypothesis represents another source of debate and controversy. Much of the data used to develop this hypothesis was collected using an animal model of concussion known as fluid percussion. In order to deliver an injury to an animal, say a mouse, by fluid percussion, the scientists perform a craniotomy, a procedure that results in the removal of a small circular portion of the mouse's skull. They connect this hole to a syringe that is half filled with a liquid, saline, and then deliver a sharp blow to the plunger of that syringe. This causes the liquid to flow through the hole in the skull increasing the pressure on the brain or percussing it. Experiments using this model of injury, fluid percussion, were conducted, while measurements of sodium and ATP were made before and after injury, leading to the hypothesis described in Chapter 2. It should be apparent to many readers, however, that concussions sustained by humans are caused by a blow to the head or other source of trauma that rapidly spins the brain. There is no hole made in the skull, no fluid percussion of the brain. It is unclear, therefore, whether or not fluid percussion is an analogous model to concussion as it occurs in life. Despite the fact that sodium ions in the ATP are clearly involved in an injury sustained by fluid percussion, it might not be the case that the same disturbances of sodium ions in ATP occur when the brain is spun rapidly. In other words, when the brain sustains a concussion, a different mechanism may be responsible for the signs and symptoms than the one described in Chapter 2; our current hypothesis may be incorrect. There remains some controversy as to whether or not this is the true biological disturbance that occurs during concussion. Indeed, although we did not discuss them in Chapter 2, there are other hypotheses being considered.

SUMMARY

There are several controversies surrounding the definition and diagnosis of concussion. Some have argued that diagnosis should only be made when there is a true, distinct, traumatic event that triggers symptoms, while others argue that the event may not be recalled by an athlete and, therefore, the diagnosis should be made when those who are at risk of sustaining a concussion suffer symptoms that are commonly associated with concussion. While the biological movement of ions and ATP that is believed to underlie the symptoms of concussion has been studied in animals, the model of injury used in those experiments is not necessarily analogous to concussions sustained by man. Therefore, debate remains as to what the true biological effects of concussion are. As the symptoms of concussion are nonspecific and currently concussion cannot be confirmed by available medical testing, some have argued the diagnostic criteria should be stricter, including not only definitive history, but also a measurable change in balance, cognition, or some other parameter besides the subjective reporting of symptoms alone. Some believe the trauma may result in a delayed onset of symptoms, while others believe that the delayed onset of symptoms is more likely to reflect a different cause of a person's symptoms than a concussion. Certainly, many of these questions could be answered more easily if there were definitive medical diagnostic tests that could be used to confirm the diagnosis of concussion. It may be that certain chemicals in the blood, urine, or saliva of athletes, or pictures of the brain such as computed tomograms or magnetic resonance images may in the future help to distinguish concussion from other entities and resolve these controversies.

CHAPTER 14

Issues Surrounding Determination of Recovery

Please recall that recovery from concussion occurs when an athlete has a full resolution of symptoms, has reachieved the baseline measures of balance, and has reachieved baseline measures of cognition. Since these domains are affected by concussion and can be measured by treating clinicians, many feel they are the best way of measuring concussions and determining recovery from concussions. They are not, however, without controversy. These criteria are subject to interpretability and, therefore, are not ideal for determining recovery from concussion.

As noted multiple times throughout this book, the symptoms of concussion are nonspecific and may be caused by other medical conditions and injuries. Furthermore, as discussed in Chapter 6, the treatment of concussion for many results in symptoms of its own. Athletes whose symptoms persist beyond the first few days or weeks can grow frustrated by the restrictions placed on their activities. Many of them may become sad and irritable about the fact that they are no longer participating in their chosen sports. As many are placed on physical rest, they are not exercising like they normally would be. Since exercise is associated with greater daytime energy, better quality sleep, and better overall mood, the lack of exercise may result in poor sleep, irritability, depression, and decreased energy. Furthermore, exercise is associated with the regulation of blood flow to the brain. When athletes, who are used to exercising regularly, suddenly stop exercising, the blood flow to the brain may become altered. This alteration in blood flow patterns may be associated with headaches, dizziness, decreased energy, and other symptoms similar to the symptoms of concussion. As many athletes are unable to complete their usual schoolwork during recovery from a concussion, they start to become anxious and emotionally stressed. This anxiety can further exacerbate their sleep disturbance and can result in headaches, difficulty sleeping, trouble concentrating, and many other symptoms similar to the symptoms of concussion. If full resolution of symptoms is used as a way of determining recovery, yet the treatments we are employing are causing some of the symptoms that we are attributing to concussion, athletes who have recovered from their concussions may be mischaracterized as still being in active recovery. Athletes, parents, and doctors may presume the athlete is still recovering from a concussion when, in actuality, the athlete has recovered, but is experiencing symptoms from a lack of exercise, poor sleep, anxiety, poorly regulated blood flow to the brain, and depression regarding the restrictions on activities, among other possible factors. Some such athletes, under the false impression that they are pushing themselves too hard, may further restrict their activities in an effort to recover faster. These athletes may fall further behind in school and grow more frustrated about their inability to participate in sports, thus making their symptoms worse, even though they have recovered from their concussions. Therefore, many have argued that full symptom resolution, when defined as no symptoms of concussion, should not be used to determine recovery. Many have argued that, given the nonspecific nature of the symptoms attributable to concussion, athletes who have not been injured may be experiencing some of these symptoms. Thus, rather than full resolution of symptoms, recovery should be determined by a substantial decrease in symptoms, placed into their proper context, and interpreted by the managing clinicians.

Furthermore, as noted in Chapter 6, some worry that athletes may report persistent symptoms in order to gain other advantages. Some may have grown accustomed to the academic accommodations that were put in place during their recovery. They may be afraid to lose those accommodations, and this fear may be exacerbated by the fact that they have fallen behind in many subjects. They may, therefore, be reluctant to give up the academic accommodations for fear it will negatively affect their school performance and, therefore, report persistent symptoms.

There is substantial controversy surrounding the use of neuropsychological assessments and computerized neurocognitive assessments for the management of sport-related concussion. Certainly, traditional neuropsychological tests that are administered and interpreted by a qualified, licensed neuropsychologist are well established within the medical tradition. These neuropsychological assessments have been used in diagnosing and managing such conditions as attention deficit hyperactivity disorder, learning disabilities, Alzheimer's disease, and stroke. In the setting of sports, in order to diagnose and assess for sport-related concussion, the use of neuropsychological assessments is relatively new. Some of the early studies surrounding this use of neuropsychological assessments were performed in the 1980s. As with symptoms, neuropsychological assessments can be affected by many factors other than concussion. Some conditions that are relatively common among athletes, such as physical fatigue, depression, viral illness, dehydration, and low motivation, among others, can affect these neuropsychological assessments. Therefore, some have argued that their role in determining recovery from concussion is limited and less important than the assessment of symptoms.

Computerized neurocognitive assessments are even more controversial than traditional neuropsychological assessments in the assessment of sport-related concussion. They are a new development, and have only been available for the last decade or two. Many have argued that they have not been studied enough to know whether or not they are accurately measuring the areas of brain function they were intended to measure. As with the traditional neuropsychological test, computerized neurocognitive assessments are also nonspecific. They may be affected by the level of effort, physical fatigue, depression, distractibility, and other factors. Furthermore, some have reported that athletes will purposely try to do poorly on the baseline measures of their computerized cognitive function so that, in the event they sustain a concussion, they will still be able to perform as well as they did on their baseline and, therefore, be allowed to continue participating in their sports even prior to full recovery. Therefore, some have argued, if too much weight is given to computerized neurocognitive tests, and some athletes are gaming the system by purposely performing poorly on their baseline, then we may risk returning them to sport too soon.

Furthermore, computerized cognitive assessments are often administered by untrained personnel. They may be administered by a neuropsychologist, which is ideal, but they may also be administered by athletic trainers, team physicians, and even nonmedical professionals. Unfortunately, they are often administered in a setting that is not conducive to optimal performance. Often, they are administered to multiple athletes at once, in a noisy and highly distractible environment. Perhaps, even less fortunately, many of those administering these tests have not been properly trained on them. If not properly trained, the assessments may be misinterpreted and, therefore, the value they add to the management and assessment of sport-related concussion—may be not only limited, but perhaps also dangerous. Take the example of the athletes who try to do poorly on their baseline assessments. Many of the computerized neurocognitive assessments have criteria that those interpreting the test can use to help determine whether an athlete has put forth a good effort. If these criteria are not met, it suggests that the athlete has purposely performed poorly. If, however, the people administering the test are not trained on how to interpret them, they may miss these criteria or be unaware they even exist. Therefore, they will not know what to check for and not recognize that the baseline is invalid. If trained properly on the interpretation of the test, the examiner will note that the test is invalid and may remove the athlete from participation until a valid test is obtained.

In addition, these tests are subject to what is known as a learning affect. Athletes who have taken the test multiple times may perform better than athletes who take the test for the first time. This is not because their cognitive function is necessarily better, but rather they have become accustomed to the test and have learned how to take it. As many of you know, the first time you are attempting to perform an activity, it often takes longer and you are less precise than if you have performed the activity multiple times over. Therefore, if athletes take the test multiple times, they may do as well as they did the first time they took it, at their baseline assessment, despite the fact that they are still injured. The learning effects from having repeated the test multiple times may compensate for the effects of injury. This, again, could result in premature return to play.

In addition, any time a person undergoes an assessment of cognitive function, their scores vary from prior tests. If you take the same test over and over again, it is unlikely that you will score exactly the same each time. Often, you get a few answers right that you answered incorrectly a previous time, or get a few answers wrong that you answered correctly the previous time. The scores are rarely exactly the same. Therefore, it is possible that some athletes who perform very well at their baseline assessment, might never perform that well again, even though they have not sustained a concussion or even if they have recovered fully from a concussion that they did sustain. This would result in prolonged restriction from activities which, as noted above, may result in symptoms in and of itself. Furthermore, if athletes are withheld from participation in sports, even when they are recovered from their injuries, they may be less likely to report injuries in the future. This could result in underreporting of concussions, a phenomenon which has already been well described.

While balance is often affected by concussions, these deficits seem to resolve quite quickly. It is rare that athletes who have sustained sport-related concussions have measurable deficits in their balance beyond the first few days after injury. Therefore, when this is used as a criterion for recovery, most athletes can reachieve their baseline balance in several days, even when other symptoms persist. If those athletes are hiding their symptoms, and balance is used as a measure of recovery, these athletes may be returned to sport too soon. Furthermore, the initial study of the balance assessments were performed using sophisticated machinery that measure postural sway, the sway back and forth that we all do when we are trying to stand still. Many athletic programs are not able to afford such expensive machinery and, therefore, use the balance error scoring system (BESS) discussed in Chapter 5. This is a rather gross assessment of balance, and athletes must have substantial deficits in their balance in order for them to be detected by this method. Therefore, many have argued that it is not sensitive enough to truly assess concussion or monitor recovery. Furthermore, the original studies showing the effectiveness of the BESS were performed by having the athlete stand on a foam pad. In reality, this test is often administered on a hard, firm surface, making it even less sensitive to the effects of concussion on balance. Therefore, many have argued this improper administration of the BESS is not ideal.

As noted above with the definition of concussion, a definitive medical test for diagnosing and measuring concussion would go a long way in helping to determine recovery.

SUMMARY

The determination of recovery from concussion is made by measuring athletes' symptoms, balance, cognitive function, and perhaps other factors. All these factors can be affected not only by concussion, but also by other factors, including effort of the athlete, motivation, dehydration, illness, anxiety, mental distraction, poor sleep, depression, among others. Many of these may result from the restrictions on activities used for the treatment of concussion. Furthermore, some believe the assessments used for measuring cognition have not been thoroughly studied and therefore, their use in clinical practice is premature, particularly when administered by those who are not properly trained. While balance is affected, sensitive measures may be needed to detect subtle changes in balance. Currently, the most widely used methods may not be sensitive enough for detecting these subtle changes in balance. In addition, athletes may downplay their symptoms and purposely perform poorly on baseline measures of cognition and balance, in an effort to return-to-play as soon as possible after injury. This phenomenon, known as underreporting of concussion, might be amplified if the measures we use for determining recovery from concussion are too restrictive, keeping athletes from participating in their sports even when they are recovered.

CHAPTER 15

Issues Surrounding Post-Concussion Syndrome

For those that sustain a concussion and experience symptoms for a long period of time, there is debate about whether or not they remain in active recovery from concussion, or whether or not they have a new baseline level of symptoms, despite the fact that they are recovered from their concussion or whether or not their symptoms are attributable to their concussion at all. It is common to read in the lay media reports of athletes who sustained a concussion and are still recovering months or even years after the injury. In the medical and scientific literature studying concussion, this is quite rare, particularly with regards to sport-related concussions. Many argue that athletes were not experiencing these symptoms prior to the time of injury, but then began to experience them at the moment of some impact to the brain or head; they continue to experience them consistently since that time and should be treated as if they have a concussion from which they are incompletely recovered. Others argue, however, that most people are susceptible to headaches and many of the other symptoms that are associated with concussion. We are fortunate in that most people, despite being susceptible to headaches, have a threshold that is fairly high and, therefore, it is only when under physical or emotional stress that they suffer headaches. Some have argued that sustaining a concussion can lower the threshold for headaches and, therefore, those who sustain a concussion are at higher risk for headaches—they suffer headaches more easily after their injury than they did previously. Therefore, the persistence of headache does not mean that they are not recovered from their concussion, but rather that they now have a lower threshold and will suffer headaches more frequently, despite the fact that they have recovered from their concussion.

Still others have noted that, since the symptoms of concussion are non-specific, they may occur due to other causes. It is, therefore, plausible that patients who suffer a concussion will attribute these symptoms, any time they experience them in the future, to their concussion. As noted above, other effects of concussion, as well as the subsequent treatment of concussion, particularly the restrictions placed on activities after a concussion, may result in symptoms of their own. These symptoms often are the same ones that result from concussion, and therefore, it can become difficult to distinguish one from the other. This further complicates the post-concussion period.

The very definition of post-concussion syndrome is controversial and often debated. Some organizations and societies define post-concussion syndrome as symptoms and signs of concussion that persist greater than three months after injury. Unfortunately, other investigators, clinicians, and scientists have defined it in various ways in the medical literature, such as the persistence of symptoms longer than two weeks, one month, or six months. This has made the study of post-concussion syndrome, its possible causes, and the best ways of treating it difficult. A population of people experiencing symptoms of concussion for longer than a week is potentially different than the population of people experiencing symptoms longer than 6 months. One can imagine that athletes who are still having symptoms 6 months after a concussion may have grown more frustrated by their lack of progress. If they are still restricted in their activities, they are more likely than athletes who are only a week out from injury to have effects from lack of exercising, falling behind at school or work, poor sleep, headaches, and other symptoms due to the restrictions placed on their activities as opposed to the concussion itself. If some or potentially all their symptoms were due to the restrictions on their activities, the treatments most likely to be effective are different than the treatments most likely to be effective for someone who is still in active recovery from a concussion. Currently, there is no test that will tell us whether or not symptoms are due to a concussion or other factors. Nor is there a test that will tell us whether someone has fully recovered from a concussion. Thus, the nature of post-concussion syndrome, what the symptoms are caused by, and how it is best managed is controversial.

Sometimes, in medicine, an injury may result in what is known as malingering. Malingering is the term used to describe someone who is exaggerating or feigning injury or illness in order to gain some benefit, such as the avoidance of work; in other words, the persistence of perpetual reporting of symptoms in order to achieve what are known as secondary gains.

As mentioned above, some athletes may grow accustomed to the academic accommodations provided to them during recovery from concussion and therefore continue to report persistent symptoms of concussion over fear of losing these academic accommodations. There are, however, other secondary gains that may result from concussion and its treatment. For example, some athletes, particularly young pediatric athletes, may not wish to participate in their sport any longer. They may not enjoy it and may, in fact, be intimidated by participation in it. In order to please their parents, coaches, teammates, and others, they may continue to participate in that sport. When they are removed from sport for treatment of their concussion, they often are pleased to be removed from the sport. Sustaining a concussion allowed them to be removed from their sport without disappointing their parents, coaches, and teammates. This may result in them reporting persistent symptoms in an effort not to return to sports without disappointing the others involved. There are still other potential secondary gains from sustaining an injury. Often, patients receive a lot of attention from their loved ones while suffering from a concussion. People go out of their way to try and help them. Some younger athletes who are so busy with sports, schoolwork, and other extracurricular activities may have limited time to spend with their parents. When they have a concussion, due to the restrictions on these activities, they may have more time to spend with their parents or on other activities they enjoy. Therefore, they malinger and continue to report symptoms in order to achieve these secondary gains.

In addition, concussion can disrupt a well-balanced, but busy, organized life. People today are under enormous pressure to achieve and be successful. Student athletes, in particular, are often involved in a highly competitive college application process. They are attempting to get straight "As" in school, excel athletically, perform well on their SATs/ACTs, and partake in many extracurricular activities, in order to set themselves apart from their peers and get accepted to a prestigious college. They operate day in and day out at maximum level, with high efficiency, making the most out of every minute of the day. When they sustain a concussion, they are often removed from school and sports for some time. This may cause them to fall behind their peers in both. If they were using all their talents and abilities to maintain their grades and athletic performance, once they fall behind, it can be very difficult to catch up. Furthermore, the thought of having to catch up and the time commitment required to do so can be overwhelming. This situation can result in emotional stress, difficulty sleeping, difficulty concentrating, and other symptoms that can be misinterpreted for the symptoms of concussion.

Summary

Post-concussion syndrome refers to the prolongation of symptoms after a concussion that exceeds some time period. The time period varies according to different definitions. It is unclear whether the persistent symptoms are due to concussion itself or other factors, including the effects of treatment for concussion, malingering, or the effects of falling behind at work, school, or in sports. As there is, as yet, no way of definitively diagnosing or measuring concussion, the causes of post-concussion syndrome are debated. Identifying the cause is important, as the treatments for the different potential causes of an athlete's symptoms vary.

CHAPTER 16

Issues Surrounding Chronic Traumatic Encephalopathy

As discussed previously, there are cumulative effects of concussion. These may be divided by time periods into immediate cumulative effects and delayed cumulative effects. The immediate cumulative effects have been studied previously. Early in the medical literature regarding concussive brain injury, a neuropsychologist, Dorothy Gronwall, measured cognitive function in patients who were referred to her clinic after sustaining a concussion. She measured their function using something called paced auditory serial addition test. During this assessment, patients were asked to listen to a list of numbers being read aloud on a cassette tape or audio file. The task is to add the most recent number that was read aloud to the previous number that was read aloud and call out the answer to the examiner. Please note, the task does not restart after every two numbers. It continues, such that once a number is called, it must immediately be added to the number that preceded it and the answer called out to the examiner. For example, if the numbers read aloud were 7, 13, 4, and 28, the examinee answering correctly would callout 20, 17, 32, and so forth. The numbers being read aloud are paced such that the answer has to be called out in sufficient time to allow the examinee to hear the next number, think of the answer, and call it out. Dr. Gronwall noticed that those patients sent to her clinic after sustaining their first lifetime concussion performed better than those who had sustained multiple lifetime concussions. Furthermore, those who were there after their first concussion seemed to return to normal values on the paced auditory serial addition test more quickly than those who were there with a repeated concussion. Therefore, Dr. Gronwall and her coinvestigator hypothesized that having sustained a previous concussion increased the duration of recovery from a recent concussion. Similar studies have been reported to confirm her findings using other forms of cognitive testing, balance assessment, duration of concussion symptoms, and even the signs of concussion noted immediately after injury. Some studies have shown that athletes who sustain a concussion are more likely to lose consciousness if they have sustained previous concussions. Furthermore, athletes who sustain a concussion are more likely to have amnesia, have a higher symptom burden, and suffer a longer duration of symptoms if they have sustained prior concussions.

Given the inability to definitively diagnose a concussion by using a standard medical test, this research, which indicated a cumulative effect of concussion, remains somewhat controversial. In the past, the diagnosis of concussion was made quite differently than it is today. There was a time when it was thought that the injury that resulted in loss of consciousness after a blow to the head was a unique and separate entity from that which resulted in dizziness, imbalance, confusion, and other symptoms that we now associate with concussion. It could be that some athletes are prone to lose consciousness when compared to others and, therefore, were more likely to be diagnosed with a previous concussion. Furthermore, many of these studies relied on the patients to report the history of previous concussion. There was no way to confirm this through footage of the sporting events, medical records, or some other means of corroborating history. Therefore, some have argued, the results are subject to what is known as recall bias. Recall bias is commonly considered when conducting medical research. As discussed in Chapter 12, recall bias stems from the fact that some people with a given injury, illness, or disease may recall previous exposures to risk factors differently than those who do not currently have an injury, illness, or disease. In this instance, it may be that those athletes who sustained a concussion that resulted in a loss of consciousness are more likely to recall having sustained previous concussions than those athletes who sustained a concussion without a loss of consciousness. This would leave the medical researcher to believe that those experiencing a loss of consciousness at the time of injury were more likely to have sustained a previous concussion than those that did not lose consciousness. In reality, it could be that both groups, those that lost consciousness and those that did not, may have the same number of previous concussions; but those who lost consciousness recall their previous injuries, while those without a loss of consciousness do not. If that were the case, there would be no cumulative effect of concussions, but investigators would erroneously conclude there was one because their studies were influenced by recall bias. It should be noted here that recall bias depends on the subject knowing whether or not they have the injury or illness in question. The problem is not that people may recall inaccurately their exposures. It is that those with a given illness to injury will recall differently than those without the injury or illness. The bias comes in to play when one group is acting differently than the other. In our example, patients that have sustained a concussion are aware that they lost consciousness, and thus, they are more likely to recall previous concussions than those who did not lose consciousness. Their recollection of previous concussions is biased by the fact that they lost consciousness with their most recent injury.

In addition to immediate cumulative effects of multiple concussions, there is also the potential for delayed cumulative effects of multiple concussions, effects which do not show up until later in life, often long after the athlete has ceased participating in sport. Several studies have suggested this. Certainly, among people who suffer major traumatic brain injuries as a result of high-force mechanism such as motor vehicle collisions, there is a body of evidence suggesting that they are at higher risk for dementia and other diseases associated with dementia such as Alzheimer's disease later in life. While there is not an association established between a single sport-related concussion and these problems, several studies suggest that sustaining multiple concussions, or multiple blows to the head even in the absence of the signs and symptoms of concussion, may increase the risk of problems later in life. One study of former players in the National Football League suggested that those who had sustained multiple concussions have a higher risk of mild cognitive impairment compared to those who sustain only one or two concussions or no concussions at all. The term cognition is a general term used to describe the processes of the mind such as thinking, concentrating, learning, reasoning, and remembering. Mild cognitive impairment for the purposes of this study was defined according to the recommendation by the American Academy of Neurology as memory complaints corroborated by a family member, objective memory problems observed by cognitive testing, in someone who has the ability to function in daily life and does not have a diagnosis of Alzheimer's disease or other form of dementia. These former football players were sent a questionnaire in which they were asked about the number of concussions they had sustained during their career/lifetime. For purposes of the study, concussion was defined as "an injury resulting from a blow to the head that caused an alteration in mental status and one or more of the following symptoms: headache, nausea, vomiting, dizziness/balance problems, fatigue, trouble sleeping, drowsiness, sensitivity to light or noise, blurred vision, difficulty remembering, and difficulty concentrating" (Guskiewicz et al. 2005). Those who reported sustaining three or more concussions were more likely to have mild cognitive impairment than those who re-ported sustaining fewer concussions. Once again, however, the results were subject to recall bias; it could be that those former NFL players, who were having memory problems, were more likely to recall previous con-cussions than those former players who were doing well without memory problems. Thus, while both groups may have sustained the same number of concussions, those with memory problems remembered their concus-sions and reported them to study investigators, while those without mem-ory problems did not remember their prior concussions.

Another population in which delayed effects of cumulative concussion were studied consisted of boxers. Starting in the early part of the 20th cen-tury, physicians noted that boxers seemed to suffer longer-term neurocog-nitive problems. Not just boxers, but one particular type of boxer known as sluggers. For those of you unfamiliar with boxing, while there are many different types of boxers, there are two broad categories in which most boxers can be placed. There are skilled boxers who, in general, are fast, ac-curate, have impeccable timing, and will beat you by out boxing you, often scoring more points by landing more punches in places for which points are awarded than their opponents. There is another broad category of box-ers known as sluggers who are not quite as skilled, quick, or accurate, but can land big, strong, powerful punches inflicting damage on their oppo-nents. Many of these boxers win by knocking their opponents down or knocking their opponents out, rendering them unconscious. Often, while they are waiting for the moment when they can land one of these big pow-erful blows, they sustain multiple punches to the head. It is in these types of boxers that physicians and researchers noted that the risk of problems later in life were highest, specifically problems with speech, memory, gait, and motor function. Often, despite not having taken any alcohol, these boxers appeared drunk to those observing them, including referees who often cancelled fights under the belief that these fighters were drunk. This appearance resulted in the term "punch-drunk syndrome" used to describe these boxers. Over time, the brains of former sluggers and other boxers were examined pathologically, in a laboratory, after the death of the box-ers. These boxers were noted to have specific patterns of abnormal protein deposits and other abnormalities of the brain that have recently come to be known as chronic traumatic encephalopathy or CTE for short. During the last decade, this type of disease pattern has been described not only in box-ers, but also in military personnel and other former professional athletes, particularly those from the National Football League. Among many, but not all of the former athletes that have these findings in their brain, their later life is characterized by memory problems, mood swings, headaches, balance problems, depression, and other psychiatric and behavioral problems, often including substance abuse. Therefore, researchers have hypothesized that there is a connection between the findings in the brain and the problems these former athletes suffer later in life.

The connection, however, between the abnormal proteins in the brain and the behavior problems observed, remains controversial. Some experts have pointed out that many patients who suffer from depression, mood problems, headaches, and other neurobehavioral problems have never played sports in which they sustained multiple concussions and do not have these abnormal findings in their brains. Therefore, they have argued, it could be that some of these former players suffer from the same problems as the rest of the population, and that it is only because they participated in football that we associate the problems with their exposure to football; we assume that their problems must be related to their exposure to football, even though many people who never played football have similar problems. Making this distinction is important for several reasons. First, if these patients are suffering from the same problems as the rest of the population, then their symptoms should be amenable to treatments, just as they are for the rest of the population. Right now, many former athletes believe their symptoms are attributable to a neurodegenerative process that began during their football careers and will continue until death. Therefore, they lose hope of any possible effective treatments. Many of them find themselves in despair. Many have committed suicide. Although we cannot determine for certain whether their suicides were due to this despair or feelings of hopelessness, certainly those feelings are unlikely to be helpful. Furthermore, many of us in medicine who spend our careers trying to care for and improve the health of athletes are trying to find ways to prevent these problems. If, in fact, the abnormal findings of the brains, in particular the hyperphosphorylated cis tau protein, are not responsible for the symptoms suffered by these former athletes, then attempts to block the formation of hyperphosphorylated cis tau will not help them. Certainly, the goal ought to be to find ways to treat chronic traumatic encephalopathy and prevent it from occurring in the first place. If we are focusing on a protein that is not the cause of the problem, we may be wasting time, effort, and money.

Lately, some argue that there is no clear evidence that trauma to the brain is what has resulted in the formation of the hyperphosphorylated cis tau, as there are no clear studies showing trauma directly resulting in this abnormal hyperphosphorylated cis tau. While this is true on a clinical level, there are animal models of repeated concussions that clearly show hyperphosphorylated cis tau results from trauma to the head and that hyperphosphorylated cis tau itself appears to be associated with at least some neurobehavioral outcomes. Still, since the mouse brain is quite different and distinct from the human brain, some have argued that this preliminary evidence is not definitive.

It is worth some further discussion here about the difference between association and causation. When variables are associated with one another, it means that the likelihood of one is more common in the presence of the other. This is a major component of studies of health using large populations—the epidemiological studies. Much of what we know about unhealthy habits and healthy habits comes from large epidemiological studies. Many of these studies follow one large group of people, known as a cohort, over time and see what behaviors and habits are associated with certain medical outcomes. There are several such well-known studies including the Framingham Heart study, the Nurses' Health Study, the Jackson Heart Study, and the Physicians' Health Study. It is from these studies that we have learned that people who smoke cigarettes are at an increased risk for lung cancer, emphysema, heart attacks, and many other health problems. Similarly, we learned that high levels of serum cholesterol, in particular one component of cholesterol known as LDL, are associated with an increased risk of heart attack and stroke. From the same studies we have learned that people who exercise regularly are at decreased risk of suffering these and many other health problems. This is an illustrative example of how the studies work with people followed over time, say a large group of nurses, and every so often they are asked to give some information about their health, their eating habits, their exercise habits, and other activities that they engage in on a regular basis. From these studies, researchers noted that people who smoked tobacco products had a much higher risk of suffering lung cancer than people who did not smoke. These studies demonstrated a clear association between smoking and the risk of suffering lung cancer. Association, however, does not necessarily mean causation. Causation would mean that smoking directly causes lung cancer and that smoking in and of itself causes lung cancer. Multiple follow-up studies were necessary to prove that smoking was not just *associated with*, but also *causative of* the increased risk of lung cancer.

Let us describe a hypothetical example where association was not directly related to causation. One can imagine that when conducting a long-term epidemiological study, researchers may have noticed that people who drank a substantial amount of alcohol during the week were at increased risk of lung cancer. It could be that people in the population who drank more than 10 alcohol-containing beverages per week were at an increased risk of lung cancer. This would establish an association between drinking alcohol and suffering lung cancer. But the alcohol may not itself have caused lung cancer. In reality, it could be that those who drank more than 10 alcohol-containing beverages per week were also more likely to smoke cigarettes. If researchers assumed that the *association* between alcohol and lung cancer was actually *causation*, they would have recommended people stop drinking alcohol beverages in order to reduce the risk of cancer. For those who stopped drinking but continued smoking, they would not have, in fact, decreased their risk of lung cancer. This would be the fault of researchers for assuming that the association was in fact causation. In this example, smoking is a confounding variable. It appeared that alcohol was associated with an increased risk of lung cancer. The investigators, however, thought that the association was between alcohol lung cancer because they neglected to account for the confounding variable of smoking. Recall from Chapter 12 that a confounding variable by definition is associated both with the predictor, in this case intake of alcohol-containing beverages, and the outcome, in this case lung cancer. Those who drank more than 10 alcohol-containing beverages per week were more likely to smoke cigarettes, and smoking is associated with an increased risk of lung cancer.

Some have argued that this same phenomenon may be taking place in the study of chronic traumatic encephalopathy. There are many other differences between the former professional football players and the general population, besides the fact that they are at increased risk of concussion. Many have argued that something to do with their genetics, there training habits, the potential use of ergogenic aids (i.e., steroids, growth hormone, creatine, among others), the way they are treated by society, changes that occur to them when they transition from a career in professional football to becoming one of the general population, or other factors may be associated with the deposition of hyperphosphorylated cis tau in the brain or possibly with the neurobehavioral outcomes they seem to suffer.

In addition, others have argued that we make assumptions that any problems former football players suffer are due to their careers in football. Much of this may be due to the attention these players receive. When a former football player commits suicide, the entire country hears about it in the newspapers, on the radio, on television, and on social media. Since we hear about former professional football players committing suicide so often, it gives us the impression that they are at particularly high risk for suicide. We thus attribute this increase risk to the fact that they participated in football, and many extrapolate even farther to assume that they must have sustained many concussions during their participation in football and that these concussions have resulted in an increased risk of suicide. It may surprise many readers to know, however, that the risk of committing suicide is higher among men in the same age group who did not play professional football than it is among those who did play professional football. When a member of the general public commits suicide, however, it does not make it into the news. Most of us never hear about it. But since we do hear about it when it is a former football player, we make the assumption that there is a particularly high risk for suicide among those who participated in American football.

SUMMARY

In summary, there is evidence suggesting that concussions can have a cumulative effect, both an immediate cumulative effect observed in the short term and a delayed cumulative effect observed more long term. As with all studies, however, the studies that illustrate this cumulative effect may be subject to recall bias, where participants aware of the outcome recall disproportionately the number of concussions they have sustained. Furthermore, there may be confounding variables that are misleading the study investigators into erroneously concluding that exposure to concussions, or even multiple blows to the head whether or not they cause concussions, are causing the problems. Finally, athletes and their issues are covered by the media to a much greater extent than the problems faced by society in general, giving many the impression that certain medical problems are more common among former NFL players, when they, in fact, may not be.

CHAPTER 17

Issues Surrounding the Role of Age and Gender

Some epidemiological studies of high school athletes have suggested that female athletes are at increased risk of sustaining sport-related concussions compared to their male counterparts, sustaining a higher number of concussions per athletic exposure. When comparing sports for which the rules are similar for female athletes as they are for male athletes, such as soccer and basketball, some studies have shown women sustain more concussions, suggesting that female athletes are at an increased risk of sustaining sport-related concussions. There are, however, many factors that differ between boys and girls that may also explain the appearance of an increased incidence of concussion. First, remember that whether or not athletes are diagnosed with a concussion relies heavily on whether athletes report their symptoms. Certainly, there are obvious concussions where athletes lose consciousness or develop gross imbalance or vomiting or some other obvious sign of concussion. Therefore, anyone on the sidelines can tell that there is something wrong and, with a little further information, can make the diagnosis of concussion. Many sport-related concussions, however, are much more subtle than that, involving some headaches, confusion, difficulty with concentration, and difficulty with memory. These injuries are more difficult to diagnose and are usually brought to attention when the athlete comes to the sidelines and reports to their athletic trainer, team physician, parents, or coach that they sustained a blow to the head resulting in symptoms. Some have argued that female athletes may simply be more honest in acknowledging their symptoms and removing themselves from play than male athletes. It may be that male athletes, perhaps due to societal pressures or expectations, may be more likely to hide their symptoms and try and push through the injury while continuing to play. Therefore, when conducting a study, one might diagnose a higher incidence of concussion among female athletes than male athletes when, in fact, the incidence may be similar, but female athletes may simply be reporting their injuries more commonly.

Similarly, other studies suggest that it takes female athletes longer to recover from sport-related concussions than male athletes. Again, the determination of recovery is often highly dependent on athletes reporting full resolution of their symptoms. Thus, it may be that female athletes are more likely to be honest about their symptoms and their symptom duration, while male athletes, possibly due to a sense of machismo or bravado, attempt to hide their symptoms from their treating clinicians in order to return to play sooner. Further confusing this picture is the fact that, in general, females tend to complain of symptoms even when they are uninjured at a higher rate than males do. In other words, females are more likely to have headaches, depression, difficulty sleeping, dizziness, and other symptoms than their male counterparts when they are uninjured. Therefore, after blow to the head, these symptoms may be interpreted as evidence of a concussion when, in fact, they represent baseline symptoms or symptoms due to other causes.

In addition to gender, the age of an athlete has been proposed as related to the incidence of concussion or the duration of symptoms. Some have argued that younger athletes are at increased risk of sustaining concussions or at increased risk of longer recovery and worse outcomes after a concussion than older athletes. Much of this thinking has been derived from the fact that studies conducted using younger athletes seem to show a longer time to recovery than studies performed on older athletes. It is very difficult, however, to compare findings across studies like that—comparing the results of one study to the results of another. Studies use different definitions of concussion, different methods of diagnosing concussion, different ways of assessing recovery from concussion, and different populations being studied, all factors that may affect the outcome of interest. Thus, the observed difference in findings may not, in fact, be due to age itself, but rather to one or more of these other factors.

For example, some studies define recovery time as the time from the date of injury until the date the athlete is cleared by a physician to return to play. Many factors, however, may affect the timing of return-to-play. It could be that physicians are simply reluctant to return younger athletes to play as soon as they are recovered from their concussions and, therefore, recommend building in extra time after their symptoms have resolved before clearing athletes to return to play. If this were the case, even if a

15-year-old athlete recovered at the same time as a nine-year-old athlete, a pediatrician may be more likely to keep the nine-year-old out of sports for an additional week or two. If return-to-play was used to define recovery in a study of young athletes, it would appear that it took the younger athletes longer to recover, when, in reality, it simply appeared the nine-year-old took longer to recover because the pediatrician exercised extra caution.

In addition, the forces involved in athletics played by older athletes are greater than those in sports played by younger athletes. This speed with which the athletes move, the forces of impact involved in the collisions, is higher among older athletes who are, in general, bigger, stronger, more coordinated, and have an improved sense of timing than younger athletes. If both younger athletes and older athletes are playing together, the older athletes may impart blows of greater force to the younger athletes. Meanwhile, older athletes themselves are absorbing blows of less force, delivered by younger, slower, weaker athletes with less precise timing. These greater forces faced by the younger athletes may result in a higher degree of injury and longer recovery times. Thus, in a study of young athletes of varying ages, it might appear that it took the younger athletes longer to recover, when, in reality, younger athletes simply sustained blows of greater force, resulting in worse injury and longer recovery times than their older counterparts.

In addition, other variables which might affect duration of recovery besides age must be considered. For example, one can imagine that athletes who are suffering from a higher burden of symptoms after injury are more likely to take longer to recover. If an athlete has simply a mild headache and some light dizziness, the athlete may recover faster than the one who has terrible headaches, terrible nausea, difficulty sleeping, difficulty with concentration, pronounced dizziness, poor memory, and many other symptoms. Therefore, if you want to know the effect of age alone, you need to compare the recovery times between those athletes of different ages that have similar symptom burdens.

There are many other such variables that one would need to control for in order to isolate out the effect of age. For example, it is well known that athletes who sustained previous concussions take longer to cover, on average, from a recent concussion than those who recently sustained their first concussion ever. Therefore, one would need to adjust for the effect of having sustained previous concussions. Similarly, if gender is associated with duration of recovery, then one would need to compare male athletes to other male athletes and female athletes to other female athletes to determine the effect of age, while simultaneously adjusting for the effect of other potential confounding variables. As you can see, it can be quite complicated to determine the precise effect of one variable, independent from all other factors. This is what makes medical research hard, and what makes the interpretation of results difficult. If investigators really want to know if there is an effect of age on recovery time, they must investigate the recovery times of patients within the same study, taken from the same population, using the same definition of concussion, the same means for monitoring recovery, and control as best as possible all other parameters that may affect recovery in order to isolate out the independent effect of age.

Other experts suggest that since the brain is still developing in young athletes, they are at higher risk for longer outcomes after concussion and therefore they should not be allowed to participate in collision sports or contact sports. Whether or not the fact that the brain is still developing in young athletes is detrimental or beneficial to someone who has sustained a concussion is unknown. There is a long-standing principle in neuroscience known as the Kennard principle, which suggests that the younger brain is more capable of adapting to injury and recovering fully from injury than the older brain. Thus, some have suggested that injuries to the brains of younger athletes may be less significant than those sustained by older athletes. Others have argued that the developing brain seems susceptible to long recovery times, since studies of athletes suggest that those who sustain concussions at a younger age are more likely to suffer problems later on. Thus, some have argued children should not be allowed to participate in sports with a high incidence of sport-related concussion.

There are, in addition, other issues that may result from delaying the age at which children can participate in contact or collision sports. As with many endeavors, it is easier to learn new skills when one is younger than it is when one is older. Many people in their forties and fifties who attempt to pick up a musical instrument find that it takes them much longer to learn the fundamentals of playing that instrument than it does for children who are able to pick up the instrument more quickly. The same is true of neuromuscular control, control of muscles and movement by the nervous system. There is an age at which children who are active athletically can develop excellent neuromuscular control. If it is not developed during that age range, it is learned only with more difficultly later in life. Since the process of delivering a blow to another athlete, or, more importantly, the process of absorbing a blow from another athlete safely, without resulting in injury, requires very precise neuromuscular control, there may be a risk to delaying participation in certain sports or certain aspects of sports such as tackling and body checking. Children who are not exposed to tackling or body checking may not develop the required skills. Thus, when they are later exposed to tackling and body checking, they may be at an increased risk of injury when compared to children with previous exposure to tackling and body checking. Indeed, there is some preliminary evidence to suggest this. A study of more than 1,500 youth ice hockey players in Canada showed that those players with previous exposure to body checking at a younger age were less likely to sustain a serious injury, resulting in more than seven days away from their sport, than those introduced to body checking for the first time at an older age (Emery et al. 2011).

Therefore, experts on all sides of the argument can be found. Some advocate delaying body checking and tackling until a certain age, usually this age is somewhere between 14 years and 15 years old, as the juvenile brain is still developing and, therefore, may be more susceptible to injury. The brain continues to develop, however, until a much later age. Thus, some argue that such an argument is at best questionable. Others argue the athletes should learn the skills required to absorb a blow or tackle when they are younger so that they can develop the necessary neuromuscular control. Furthermore, the speed and forces involved in collisions sustained by young athletes are much lower than their older counterparts. Thus, some have argued, it is better to learn those skills when young and when the forces involved are less harmful than they are at an older age. Perhaps, a reasonable compromise, some argue, is to teach the skills to young athletes in a controlled setting, where the risk of injury is minimal.

SUMMARY

In summary, some studies suggest that both age and gender affect the risk of sport-related concussion and the duration of recovery from sport-related concussion. It can be hard, however, to isolate the independent effect of each of the factors, as many other factors play a role in the risk of injury and the duration of recovery. It can be difficult to compare across studies, as each medical study is conducted differently, using different definitions, different methods for measuring, and using different populations. Despite these limitations, some have called for the delaying of tackling and body checking until a certain age. Such a delay may not be without risk, and, therefore, others have argued no such change in the current rules is warranted.

CHAPTER 18

Issues Surrounding Neuropsychological/ Neurocognitive Assessments

The role of neuropsychological and neurocognitive testing in the assessment and management of sport-related concussion is controversial. But, before we discuss the controversy, it is worth making a distinction between neuropsychological testing and computerized neurocognitive testing. In general, neuropsychological testing involves measurements of patients' mental status, cognitive function, social well-being, and other assessments made by a trained neuropsychologist who has either a Doctorate of Philosophy (PhD) or a Doctorate of Psychology (PsyD) with specific training in measuring the functions of the mind and interpreting variables that affect the function of the mind. Neurocognitive testing is a more limited assessment of cognition and symptoms of a person made by administering computerized assessments but without formal evaluation by a neuropsychologist.

Please recall that for a long time the diagnosis of concussion was made solely on the basis of visible signs of injury and the symptoms experienced by the athletes. During the 1980s, and particular during the 1990s and early 2000s, neuropsychologists began evaluating the effects of concussion on brain function. In a series of studies, it was revealed that concussion was associated with decreases in cognitive functioning including reaction time, memory, the ability to concentrate, the speed with which information was processed, and other functions. In fact, among a substantial proportion of athletes that had sustained sport-related concussions, these deficits in cognition persisted even after the athlete reported symptom resolution. Therefore, many argue that neuropsychological testing or computerized neurocognitive testing offers an objective means of monitoring recovery and offers additional information as to the status of the athlete that has sustained a concussion in addition to what can be gleaned from monitoring symptoms alone.

The issue remains controversial, however, as both formal neuropsychological testing and neurocognitive testing are affected by many factors. The assessment is not black or white and does not answer definitively whether an athlete has sustained a concussion or not. Nor do these assessments definitively determine whether an athlete who is known to have sustained a concussion has recovered or not. Neurocognitive function can be affected by many other factors besides concussion such as depression, motivation, changes in sleep pattern, fatigue, mood, anxiety, illness, poor nutrition, and many other factors. While neuropsychological evaluation by a neuropsychologist can be more useful in determining these factors and interpreting the findings, there still remains a substantial amount of ambiguity. In fact, even among uninjured athletes, test performance varies between tests taken at different times; uninjured athletes tested on more than one occasion score differently each time the test is taken. These limitations are compounded when neurocognitive testing is used without a neuropsychologist or other clinician properly trained in the use of such tests.

Thus, many experts argue that the testing should be used on athletes and offers some additional information that will help a clinician ultimately make the diagnoses and ultimately determine recovery when added to the other components of the evaluation. Others argue that, given the lack of specificity of these tests and their variability even among uninjured athletes, they should not be used at all.

Regardless of the controversy about whether or not these tests should be used, all experts agree that, if these tests are used, they should not be used in isolation to determine whether or not an athlete has recovered, but rather as an additional part of the clinical picture helping to determine recovery.

Even among those who agree that the tests are useful for athletes at risk of sustaining sport-related concussions, there is some controversy as to whether or not baseline evaluations are necessary and should be mandatory for athletes, particularly those in high-risk sports such as football, soccer, lacrosse, ice hockey, and field hockey, among others. Many people argue that there is a high degree of variability in the athletic population with regards to cognition. Some athletes have impeccable memory, while others struggle with memory. This is true of the general nonathletic population as well. Given this high degree of variability, some argue, that without baseline testing, many scores would be difficult to interpret. For example, if an athlete has sustained a sport-related concussion and several days later reports being completely symptom free, including with full non-risk, noncontact exercise, one might administer a computerized neurocognitive test as a means of gaining further information to determine whether or not the athlete is fully recovered and may return to contact sports. One can imagine that such an athlete might score in the 60th percentile with regards to memory, meaning that the athlete's memory is better than 60 percent of those taking the test, but not as good as 40 percent of those taking the test. Without a baseline assessment, it is difficult to know whether the 60th percentile represents recovery or not. One can imagine that athletes with impeccable memories may score in the 95th percentile when they are uninjured, and that the 60th percentile represents a significant decrease from their baseline abilities, indicating that they are not yet recovered. On the other hand, many athletes will score at the 60th percentile at baseline when they are uninjured, and therefore, this score of 60th percentile after injury does represent recovery. Without a baseline score, taken when an athlete is uninjured, it can be difficult to interpret; by itself, the 60th percentile can represent injury or recovery, depending on the athlete's pre-injury capabilities. Thus, many have argued that baseline testing should be obtained on all athletes in sports with a significant risk of sport-related concussion.

Note that deficits in neurocognitive scores are nonspecific in nature. One can imagine that athletes who took their baseline in August and did quite well may have other factors affecting their scores when they sustain a concussion, say in November. If such an athlete has just broken up with his girlfriend, he may not been sleeping well and may be saddened by his recent breakup. Perhaps, he has difficulty concentrating, as his mind is preoccupied with the break up and, therefore, his grades have suffered. Anxiety over the decrease in his grades and his future success when applying to college may be keeping him awake at night. Even when he recovers from his injury, the depression, anxiety, lack of sleep, and difficulty concentrating may result in decreased neurocognitive test scores. He may be then held out of sports, despite the fact that he has recovered from his concussion, as his decrease in test scores may be interpreted as incomplete recovery. This restriction from athletic activity may only worsen his depression, thereby exacerbating and prolonging his symptoms. Many argue that it is due to situations like this that there is no role for neurocognitive testing in the management of sport-related concussion, particularly when administered by those who are not properly trained to interpret them.

Still others argue that, in addition to the role in helping with diagnosis and monitoring recovery, neurocognitive assessments play a role in prognosis from concussion, in estimating when an athlete is likely to be recovered. Athletes who score well on these assessments after sport-related concussion are likely to recover in a shorter period of time than those who score markedly worse than their own personal baseline assessments. Therefore, the test may be useful in planning the overall treatments, planning for a prolonged absence from sports, and planning to make accommodations for athletes who are in school or employed during recovery. If they score poorly, preparations can be made for a possible long recovery. Others argue that such planning and accommodations can be made even in the absence of computerized neurocognitive and neuropsychological assessments.

Among those who believe these assessments are useful, there is controversy surrounding which types of test are most appropriate. Some neuropsychologists feel that formal neuropsychological assessment by a trained and licensed neuropsychologist is the only way to properly assess brain function, either at baseline or after a sport-related concussion. Some argue that one cannot train on these assessments without undergoing the formal and official training required for a doctoral degree and licensure. Still others argue that there are not enough neuropsychologists to perform baseline or postinjury assessments on all the athletes who engage in sports where concussions occur commonly. This is particularly true for more rural settings were neuropsychologists are rare. In addition, the assessments performed to inform sport-related concussion represent only a limited part of neuropsychology and can be learned without studying the entire field of neuropsychology. Finally, neuropsychologists and formal neuropsychological evaluation is lengthy, expensive, and would be cost prohibitive if required for all athletes engaged in contact sports, collision sports, and other sports during which concussions occur so commonly. Therefore, many argue, neurocognitive testing by those trained just on the computerized neurocognitive assessment opposed to the entire field of neuropsychology add valuable information, are comparatively inexpensive, take less time, allowing for the simultaneous testing of multiple athletes once, making them that much more feasible.

SUMMARY

In summary, the role of neuropsychological and neurocognitive testing in the assessment and management of sport-related concussion is controversial. Some argue that neuropsychological testing or computerized neurocognitive testing offers additional objective information for diagnosing concussion and monitoring recovery above the reporting and monitoring of symptoms alone. As the assessments are nonspecific and variable, even among uninjured athletes that undergo repeated testing, some argue there is currently no role for such assessments in the management of sport-related concussion. Even among those in favor of their use, whether formal neuropsychological evaluation with a neuropsychologist is necessary or whether computerized neurocognitive measures suffice, is hotly debated. Regardless of these debates, all experts agree that, if these tests are used, they should not be used in isolation to determine whether or not an athlete is recovered, but rather as an additional part of the clinical picture helping to determine recovery.

CHAPTER 19

Issues Surrounding Treatment of Concussion

Treatment of concussion itself is somewhat controversial. Most expert guidelines recommend that sport-related concussions be treated with rest—both physical and cognitive rest. Physical rest is relatively understood by most athletes. It involves removing them from vigorous physical exercise and training. One benefit of removal from play is that it removes athletes from the risk of additional blows to the head, which are more common during practice and gameplay than they are in the activities of everyday life. This allows the brain to recover without sustaining additional insult. Furthermore, if energy is required, in the form of ATP, for the brain to heal from a concussion, then engaging in physical exercise would have the effect of stealing ATP away from the brain and putting it toward the skeletal muscles. This would only exacerbate the underlying problem. Therefore, physical rest also results in conservation of energy that can be applied toward the healing brain. Cognitive rest is a little more complicated and not quite as readily understood by most, although the same principles apply. While reading a book or playing a videogame or engaging in other activities that demand concentration, focus, memory, reasoning, and attention do not cause a person to breathe heavily and sweat, they still require a substantial amount of ATP. Therefore, by restricting these activities, one will be conserving ATP, making it available to the brain for the healing process. It is for these reasons, mainly, that most expert guidelines and recommendations suggest both physical and cognitive rest after concussion. Initially, it was recommended that physical and cognitive rest be used until symptoms resolve. Once athletes became symptom free, it was recommended that they gradually be allowed to return to physical and cognitive activity as tolerated. If their symptoms recurred after they began exercising or engaging in increased cognitive activity, they would again be put to rest for a day or two and then attempted to progress again. Since most athletes recover from their concussions quickly, in a matter of a few days to a week, this was an effective strategy for most sport-related concussions.

There are, however, many athletes who suffer symptoms of concussion for longer than a few days or a week. The value of continuing to recommend physical and cognitive rest in that setting is less clear. Expert guidelines still maintain that this should be continued until full resolution of symptoms. However, many studies over the last few years have suggested that the restriction of activities, both physical and cognitive, is associated with symptoms of its own, particularly for younger athletes. When they are removed from their sports, removed from some if not all of their classes at school, it produces a certain amount of anxiety in younger athletes. They lose some of their identity, as they are no longer identified as part of their sports team. They are not getting regular exercise and, as a result, often have difficulty sleeping at night. Those who exercise regularly burn off energy during the day, which helps them sleep at night. In addition, those who exercise regularly have more energy throughout the day. Athletes restricted from exercising may lose these benefits, resulting in decreased energy throughout the day and difficulty sleeping at night. Since trouble sleeping and low energy are also symptoms of concussion, many of the clinicians treating these athletes will assume that their symptoms are due to incomplete recovery from concussion when in fact they may be the result of the restrictions on physical activity, the treatment that was designed to treat their concussion. In addition, the sudden cessation of physical activity may change the regulation of blood flow to the brain. Blood flow to the brain becomes less effective. Upsetting the normal regulation of blood flow to the brain is associated with dizziness, headaches, fatigue, difficulty concentrating, and many other symptoms, often attributable to a concussion.

Restriction of cognitive activity beyond the first few days may also have downsides. The restriction from cognitive activity may result in many athletes not performing all their required homework assignments, tests, and quizzes. This causes them to fall behind in their subjects. They are aware that, once they are recovered, they will have to take all the tests and quizzes they postponed and perform all the missed homework assignments. As these assignments and tests pile up, it can cause a substantial amount of anxiety as athletes begin to wonder how they will ever be able to makeup so much work when they recover from their concussions and return to school. This anxiety itself is associated with symptoms such as trouble concentrating, difficulty sleeping at night, fatigue during the day, headaches, nausea, and other symptoms that are often attributable to concussion. This too can lead the treating clinician to believe the symptoms are due to a concussion from which the athlete is not yet recovered. This may lead to further restrictions in activity. Further restriction may only exacerbate the problem, leading to a cycle of worsening symptoms, followed by more restrictions, followed by worsening symptoms, all under the mistaken notion that the symptoms are due to incomplete recovery from a concussion.

Several studies have shown that when you restrict the activities of adolescent athletes, even in the absence of a concussion, they go on to develop symptoms nearly identical to those that are sustained by athletes with concussion. Therefore, some of the symptoms athletes suffer after concussion, particularly those who do not resolve over the first few days, may be attributable to the treatment recommendations as opposed to the underlying process of concussion itself. In one study of patients cared for in the emergency department after a concussion, some were recommended to a few days of rest followed by gradual resumption of their activities, while others were recommended to a longer period of strict rest. Those who were allowed to resume their activities gradually after a few days of rest did better on most outcomes than those who were recommended longer periods of strict rest. Therefore, controversy exists about the proper use of rest after concussion, and the optimal duration of rest that should be recommended.

For those whose symptoms are prolonged, some physicians will use medications to treat the symptoms of concussion. Many of these medications are commonly used for the treatment of other conditions. For example, athletes who sustain a sport-related concussion that is associated with headaches are often given medications to treat those headaches. Preventative headache medications are known to decrease the intensity and frequency of headaches suffered by those in the general population. They have not, however, been studied thoroughly in the setting of sport-related concussion. Therefore, their effectiveness in this particular population remains unknown. As such, some argue that athletes with headaches from a sport-related concussion should not be treated with headache prevention medications. Other argue, however, that a headache is a debilitating symptom, and since there are effective treatments for headaches they should be employed regardless of the cause of the headaches.

The same can be said for medications treating other symptoms. Those athletes who have prolonged difficulties with memory, problems with concentration, and decreased energy levels after sustaining a sport-related concussion might benefit from stimulant medications such as those used for patients with attention deficit hyperactivity disorder, commonly abbreviated to ADHD. While these medications are frequently used and have been studied for use of problems like attention deficit hyperactivity disorder, they have not been thoroughly studied in the setting of concussion and sport-related concussion in particular. Therefore, many argue they should not be used in this setting. Others argue, since these medications can improve concentration, memory, and daytime energy, they should be considered for use in athletes with a sport-related concussion who are suffering from prolonged symptoms of this nature.

As always, when considering the use of a prescription medication, doctors will consider the potential negative effects of that medication. All medications have side effects. Some of those may be beneficial, but others can be harmful. As many athletes have difficulty sleeping after sustaining a sport-related concussion, when symptoms persist, doctors often consider treating this insomnia with medication. Fortunately, there are many effective treatments for difficulty sleeping. Some of them do not involve medication at all; rather, they start with what is known as sleep hygiene, recommendations for habits surrounding bedtime and sleep time that help achieve optimal sleep. This is particularly important in the modern age of electronics and technology. Many athletes are constantly using mobile phones, computer screens, televisions, video games, and other such products associated with bright lights, and in particular what is known as the blue light. It turns out that exposure to blue light, the type of light that is produced by phone, television, and computer screens, can suppress a natural hormone released by the brain known as melatonin. Melatonin is associated with sleepiness. One of the reasons that we get sleepy at night is that darkness and lowering of the temperature increases the secretion of melatonin into the bloodstream. The melatonin results in us feeling sleepy. If the release of melatonin is suppressed by blue light, then athletes struggling with insomnia after a sport-related concussion will be better off avoiding these types of screens an hour or more prior to their bedtime, in order to allow the natural release of melatonin into the bloodstream and help make them sleepy. Furthermore, the constant access to mobile phones provides constant communication and stimulation. Athletes should consider putting phones, televisions, computer screens, and other such devices outside the bedroom. It is difficult to sleep when your cell phone keeps vibrating, pinging, or ringing, alerting you that you have a message from one of your friends. The temptation to pick it up, look at the message, and respond is too great. Of course, once you turn on the device and look at the screen, the blue light suppresses melatonin, thereby making it even more difficult to return to sleep. Furthermore, these devices often serve as a reminder of all the tasks one needs to complete the following day. Even such things as bags, briefcases, and daily schedules can be a reminder of all the things that lie ahead the following day. Anxiety over those tasks can also make it more difficult to fall asleep. Therefore, the room in which an athlete who has sustained a concussion wishes to sleep should be dark, quiet, without any of these potential stimulators, screens, or other reminders of the following day's duties.

Since melatonin is an endogenous hormone produced by the brain, it is also a safe medication that one might take, if they are still having difficulty sleeping even after employing proper sleep hygiene. As it is a naturally occurring hormone, it is really not associated with significant side effects when taken in the recommended dosages.

There are other medications that are effective at helping athletes sleep after a concussion that are prescribed by doctors. Some of these, however, are associated with significant side effects and must be considered carefully prior to their use. While the use of sleep hygiene and melatonin results in little controversy after a concussion, the use of these other medications, some of which can suppress cognition as a side effect, generates more debate.

SUMMARY

In summary, the treatment of concussion is unsettled and currently in the midst of vigorous debate. While most experts recommend some physical and cognitive rest after injury, the recommendation for rest is not universal. Among those who do recommend rest after injury, the degree of rest, the specific restrictions recommended, and the duration of optimal rest represent an active area of controversy. While many clinicians use medications to treat some of the more common symptoms of concussion, few of these medications have been thoroughly studied for use treating concussions. Therefore, some experts recommend against their routine use.

CHAPTER 20

Issues Surrounding Second Impact Syndrome

One reason why clinicians recommend athletes suffering from the symptoms of sport-related concussion do not return to their sport is the risk of the devastating neurological injury known as second impact syndrome. The original case of second impact syndrome was described by Doctors Saunders and Harbaugh in 1984. They described the case of a collegiate football player who sustained a concussion during a physical altercation with another male. He returned to football practice a few days later while still complaining of a headache, albeit a mild headache, from his concussion. As was common practice at the time, he was permitted to return to play. He did not sustain any major traumas or injuries that were noticed by the other players or coaching staff, but at one point, he walked off the field and fell unconscious. He was taken to a local hospital where he underwent heroic measures in an attempt to save his life. Unfortunately, despite these efforts, he died. At autopsy, he was found to have massive swelling of the brain and changes associated with decreased blood flow to the brain and a lack of oxygen delivery to the brain. Doctors Saunders and Harbaugh hypothesized that, perhaps, since he had not yet recovered fully from his concussion, he was predisposed to the massive swelling of the brain, decreased blood flow, and decreased oxygen delivery that ultimately resulted in his death.

Since its original description by Saunders and Harbaugh up to the present day, the topic of second impact syndrome has been entrenched in controversy, with some questioning whether or not such a syndrome exists. It has been well established for years that trauma to the brain can result in swelling of the brain and death. This happens after a single blow to the

head, without preexisting concussion. This is particularly true in the pediatric and adolescent age group. Therefore, many authors argue that no
initial concussion is required. The injury is a result of brain trauma, not
necessarily one that was preceded by a concussion from which the athlete
was incompletely covered. Perhaps, they argue, the preexisting concussion sustained by the athlete described by Saunders and Harbaugh was
inconsequential; even had he not sustained that injury, he would have met
the same fate. Or, perhaps, the injury was never a concussion, but rather
a more severe injury which led to swelling and death four days later, and
that this would have occurred even if he did not report to football practice
that day.

There have, however, been several similar cases reported over the last
30 years, where athletes have sustained minor trauma while recovering
from a sport-related concussion, and developed massive swelling of the
brain leading to their death. Prior concussions have been documented
within a month of the injury that ultimately resulted in brain swelling and
death of many athletes. Thus, those who believe in second impact syndrome, who believe that while in recovery from a concussion the brain
is in a vulnerable state wherein an additional impact to the head, even a
minor one, may result in brain swelling and death, argue that it would be
too coincidental for so many cases of brain swelling and death to have
been preceded by a concussion. Furthermore, some researchers have been
able to re-create this phenomenon in the laboratory using animal models
of brain injury. This evidence suggests that something about the initial
injury predisposes the brain to swelling, which ultimately leads to death.
While all acknowledge that there are cases of a single blow to the head
causing brain swelling and death in the absence of a preexisting concussion, usually these injuries are caused by a more severe, forceful blow to
the head than typically occurs during sports and have typically been reported in cases of second impact syndrome.

Those who argue against the existence of second impact syndrome,
who believe that the initial injury is not required for a blow to the head to
result in brain swelling in death, point out that brain swelling and death
from a blow to the head in the absence of concussion is a well-described
phenomenon. They further point out that, in many of the cases that have
been described as second impact syndrome, it was unknown that the athletes had sustained prior concussions until after their deaths. At that point,
clinicians, researchers, or others went back and asked friends and family
members of the athletes whether or not he had sustained a prior concussion. While in each case someone recalled a prior blow to the head or
that the athlete was complaining of some symptoms prior to the injury,

concussions are common among athletes participating in the sports that have resulted in these cases being described as second impact syndrome. Therefore, if you randomly sampled a group of athletes participating in these sports, many would recall having sustained a concussion in the past. Furthermore, the symptoms of concussion are nonspecific and common, they can be caused by or result from many other conditions besides concussion, some of which have been described earlier in this book, including lack of sleep, anxiety, depression, viral illness, lack of exercise, emotional stress, dehydration, and many others. Therefore, if you were to randomly sample a group of athletes and ask them about these symptoms, many would report the symptoms even in the absence of a concussion. Thus, some experts have argued that after the death has occurred, going back and finding out that some of these athletes had sustained previous concussions or were suffering from some of these symptoms does not necessarily mean that the concussion predisposed them to brain swelling and death. Perhaps, these athletes sustained a single blow to the head that resulted in their death, and given how common they are, had some vague symptoms that were not due to a concussion or sustained some minor blow to the head that did not result in a concussion.

AGE AND GENDER

Nearly all the cases of second impact syndrome described in medical literature involve a young, male athlete, usually a teenager or young adult. This has led to the belief that second impact syndrome is an injury particular to young, male athletes and not a concern for older athletes or female athletes. There are, however, cases that appear to be second impact syndrome that have occurred in female athletes, but have not been described in the medical literature. Furthermore, given the frequency of collisions to the head during sports that predispose athletes to either concussion or second impact syndrome, most are played by young men. Outside of professional football, it is unusual to see men in their thirties and forties playing full-collision tackle football. Very few women play tackle football. Women and older men are also less commonly involved in boxing, another sport in which cases of second impact syndrome have been described. Therefore, the athletes most involved in the sports in which second impact syndrome has been described are young, often the age of junior high school, high school, or college students. Thus, there are few older men and few women at risk for second impact syndrome. Since second impact syndrome is rare, with only a handful of cases described each year, it is not surprising that it has not yet been described in female athletes or older male athletes. Thus, the role of age and gender in the development of second impact syndrome remains a source of debate and discussion among specialists.

SUMMARY

In summary, second impact syndrome is the term used to describe a phenomenon, where an athlete who is still recovering from a sport-related concussion sustains a second blow to the head, often a minor blow, and develops massive brain swelling, ultimately causing the athlete's death. Several such cases have been described in the medical literature. Some have argued that, because a single injury can result in brain swelling and concussions are so common in sports, there may be no such thing as second impact syndrome. Rather, a single blow to the head may be causing the brain swelling, without a prior concussion; any evidence of prior concussion is circumstantial or coincidental. While it appears to occur most commonly among young, male athletes, leading to the belief that second impact syndrome is an injury particular to young men, it could simply be that young men participate in the sports that carry the highest risk of concussion and second impact syndrome, and that if women or older men participated in these sports at the same rate as young men, they would suffer the injury just as often.

CHAPTER 21

Issues Surrounding Heading in Soccer

Concussion results from rapid rotational acceleration of the brain: This is often due to trauma, a direct blow to the head itself. Therefore, efforts have been made to eliminate blows to the head that occur during sports. Soccer is a relatively unique sport, in that the athlete purposefully uses his or her head to move the soccer ball. When the soccer ball is up in the air, athletes will purposefully arch their back and neck in a windup maneuver, and then forcefully strike the ball with their foreheads in order to direct the ball to another player or into the net. Some people, particularly parents of young soccer players, have worried that this purposeful heading may itself be harmful. Thus, they have argued for banning purposeful heading of the ball from soccer. They argue that if being struck in the head leads to concussion, then repeatedly striking the ball with the head must cause concussion. There are, however, large medical studies which have recorded all the concussions that have occurred during soccer tournaments; none have occurred from purposeful heading of the soccer ball. Therefore, others argue that since purposeful heading of the soccer ball does not appear to be causing a significant number of concussions, if any, there is no need to ban it from the game of soccer.

Still, purposeful heading of the ball does not occur in isolation. Many times, when a soccer player jumps into the air with the intent of heading the ball, there is another, opposing player coming from the other direction who also intends to head the ball. Many times, the two players collide. Sometimes, one is struck in the head by the opponent and sustains a concussion. Often, the collision throws one or both the players off balance and they may strike their heads on the ground when they land, resulting in a concussion. Sometimes, as an offensive player attempts to head the ball into the net, particularly on corner kicks, the opposing goalie charges out of the net, fists first, in an attempt to punch the ball away. Goalies can collide with the offensive player in these situations and cause a concussion. Therefore, while purposeful heading of the ball seems to be an uncommon cause of sport-related concussion, being in the process of heading the ball is a high-risk situation that may result in concussion. Therefore, some have argued that for this reason alone, purposeful heading of the soccer ball ought to be banned. Others have recommended that, if it is not banned for the entire sport of soccer, it ought to be banned in youth soccer.

Even if purposeful heading of the soccer ball does not result in a sport-related concussion, some worry about the potential for cumulative effects of multiple subconcussive blows—blows to the head that do not cause the signs or symptoms necessary for making the diagnosis of concussion. Please recall that in the chapter regarding chronic traumatic encephalopathy, one hypothesis considered the possibility that it is not just multiple concussions that can result in chronic traumatic encephalopathy, but possibly the accumulation of blows to the head over the course of a career whether or not they result in the signs and symptoms of concussion—subconcussive blows. If this is true, some argue, then repeated heading of the soccer ball would constitute a substantial number of subconcussive blows and, therefore, increase the risk of chronic traumatic encephalopathy. Therefore, heading should be banned.

Please recall it is the acceleration, in particular the rotational acceleration, of the brain which results in concussion. Some argue that if subconcussive blows have an effect on the brain, it likely results from this same mechanism, that is, rotational acceleration. In sports, like American football or ice hockey, the head is constantly being struck and accelerated by collisions with other athletes, the ice, the dasher boards, the field, or other structures. These collisions involve some rotational acceleration of the head, even in the absence of the signs and symptoms of concussion. Heading a soccer ball, however, results in minimal rotational acceleration of the brain. The athlete is purposely striking the ball. Using proper technique, athletes arch their back and neck and drive the mass of their body and head forward, contracting the muscles as they do so. Given the overall mass and strength of the athletes involved, and the relatively small mass of the soccer ball, the acceleration of the ball after impact is much greater than any acceleration of the athlete's head. Therefore, many have argued, there is unlikely to be any significant effect on health or brain structure as a result of purposeful heading.

Medical studies have been undertaken to try to inform the debate. Some have shown differences between the brains of soccer player who frequently head the ball and those who do not frequently head the ball on images taken by doctors known as magnetic resonance images. Thus, those in favor of banning purposeful heading of the ball argue these images are evidence of brain damage. There are, however, several limitations to these studies. First, whether or not there are differences in brain images is less important than signs or symptoms to most athletes. The differences in images are not necessarily damaging, but simply differences. If the brains look different, but the players feel well and have no problems, the significance of the images is unclear. In fact, it may be that there are differences between the brains of athletes that occur due to many other things that nobody has bothered to study, such as genetics, caffeine use, alcohol use, the use of specific nutrients, or many other things. Furthermore, it is possible, perhaps even likely that these differences in brain images are due to concussions as opposed to sub-concussive blows from purposeful heading of the ball. As described above, the act of purposeful heading is a high-risk situation for sustaining a concussion. Therefore, those players who frequently head the ball are at higher risk for sustaining concussions than those who head the ball less frequently. The differences in brain images, therefore, may be because those who frequently head the ball sustained a higher number of concussions.

Other investigators have examined the effect of heading on neurocognitive assessment. Some studies have shown a difference in neurocognitive and neuropsychological test scores between those players who report frequently heading the ball and those who do not frequently head the ball. As with imaging, however, it is likely that those who have frequently headed the ball have also sustained a higher number of concussions, and that it is the concussions that have been linked to the poorer performance on neurocognitive measures. Furthermore, other studies show no difference in performance on these assessments, calling into question the potential effect of heading the soccer ball. Given what we have learned previously about recall bias and the high rates of underreporting concussions by athletes, these studies are difficult to conduct and drawing accurate conclusions from them is even more difficult.

SUMMARY

In summary, the concern over sport-related concussion has led to further discussion about purposeful heading of the ball in soccer. While heading of the ball itself is an uncommon cause of concussion, athletes that are in the act of heading a ball are vulnerable to collisions that may cause concussions. In addition, some worry about the potential for long-term effects from purposeful heading of the soccer ball. As there are scant, limited data regarding the potential effects from purposeful heading of the ball, there is substantial controversy surrounding potential rule changes to the game that would call for a ban on the act of purposeful heading.

CHAPTER 22

Issues Surrounding the Medical Ethics of Participation in Sports

In order to more thoroughly discuss the medical ethics surrounding participation in sports, we need to briefly discuss some of the underlying principles that make up the foundation of much of modern-day medical ethics. While a thorough discussion of the principles of biomedical ethics is not appropriate for this text, some basic understanding is required to facilitate the discussion.

There are four main clusters of principles commonly used in modern-day medical ethics, each of which will be discussed further below:

1) Respect for autonomy, respect for the decision-making capabilities of a person
2) Nonmaleficence, the avoidance of causing harm
3) Beneficence, ensuring benefits to the person involved
4) Justice, ensuring that the benefits and risks involved are distributed fairly

RESPECT FOR AUTONOMY

The principle of respect for autonomy acknowledges and confirms the right of a person to make choices and to take actions independently, based on their own personal values and their own personal beliefs. In the United States and many other Western cultures, this principle is a very strong culturally held belief, crucial to us, and the basis for our modern-day systems of governing and politics. It is derived, in part, from the philosophical teachings of Immanuel Kant and John Stuart Mill, which have influenced much of American and European civilization. In sports, the respect for autonomy has been emphasized in the codes of ethics of the International Federation of Sports Medicine, which explicitly states: "The team physician must . . . not refuse an athlete the right to make their [sic] own medical decisions." In addition, the code of ethics of the American Medical Association also confirms this respect for autonomy with regards to athletes by explicitly stating, "Physicians should assist athletes to make informed decisions about their participation in amateur and professional contact sports which entail risks of bodily injury." In brief, the respect for autonomy requires us to allow athletes who are informed about the risks and benefits of participation in their chosen sports, and who are acting intentionally and without controlling influences from other parties, to decide for themselves whether or not they wish to participate.

NONMALEFICENCE

The principle of nonmaleficence emphasizes an obligation to avoid inflicting harm intentionally. This principle is a strong foundation in the medical tradition that was underscored by Hippocrates, one of the founding fathers of modern-day medicine, and is expressed in the Hippocratic oath taken by physicians as, "I will use treatment to help the sick according to my ability and judgment, but I will never use it to injure or wrong them" (Beauchamp and Childress 1994). Thus, when acting as a physician providing medical care to an athlete and deciding whether or not the athlete should be allowed to participate in sports, the principle of nonmaleficence dictates that we should avoid the causation of intentional harm.

BENEFICENCE

The principle of beneficence mandates us to provide benefits to the athletes we care for; it represents a moral obligation to act for the benefit of the athletes under our charge and in our care. As such, it requires us to allow athletes to participate in sports, and thereby derive the benefits of sports participation, unless there is just cause compelling us to act otherwise.

JUSTICE

Last, the principle of justice underscores the need for fairness and equity in the distribution of goods, benefits, the avoidance of harm, and other valuable assets. The principle of justice mandates that we are fair, using just procedures to make our decisions, and writing just policies that regulate participation in sports and that result in just outcomes, such as the equal distribution of the potential benefits to all.

Ethical principles are neither universal nor absolute. Principles require balancing and interpretation. Indeed, ethical principles often come into conflict with one another. In such circumstances, a moral and ethically sound action can only be determined by balancing one principle against the other. As an example, let us discuss a common scenario involving the decision to have surgery or not. Surgery is, in fact, a form of harm for patients. It is trauma, albeit a very controlled, purposeful, and directed trauma. Nonetheless, it is a form of trauma. If a patient has severe osteoarthritis (inflammation of the joints) of the knee, there is a decision to be made: should the knee joint be surgically replaced or not. The principle of nonmaleficence mandates that our treatments do no harm to the patient. In order to replace the knee, the surgeon must cut through the skin, dissecting many of the underlying soft tissues, break multiple bones, and replace them with artificial products, and then try to repair all the damage just caused. Indeed, even when perfectly and properly performed, there are risks involved in surgery, such as infection of the tissues, allergic reactions to anesthesia, and even, although rarely, death. Therefore, the principle nonmaleficence suggests we should not subject anyone to these harms and potential risks. The principle of beneficence, however, mandates that we must act to benefit our patients. Therefore, we should recognize that replacing the knee joint would allow patients to return to the activities of daily living and other activities they enjoy, such as regular exercise, in a pain-free manner. As neither of these principles is universal nor absolute, we must weigh the benefits against the risks and determine which takes precedence. Since the risk of allergic reaction to anesthesia, and death are minimal, and the trauma caused by surgery is directed, limited, and purposeful and the potential benefits to patients with severe arthritis is substantial in that they may return to a pain-free life and return to the activities that they most enjoy, the benefits of joint replacement surgery outweigh the risks for many patients. Therefore, the principle of beneficence should be given more weight than that of nonmaleficence in this scenario. Please note that this is not universal and this balance may change. For patients that have relatively mild osteoarthritis, they might also derive some benefit from joint replacement, but that mild benefit may not outweigh the risks involved with surgery. Therefore, the principle of beneficence would take priority over nonmaleficence. In that situation, we would not recommend joint replacement but rather one of the alternative therapies that have lower risks of harm.

In sports medicine, it is quite common that ethical principles come into conflict. All sports involve a risk of sport-related injuries. The risks of injuries of certain sports are very low, while in other sports they are higher. Sport-related concussion is a relatively common injury sustained by athletes, but is fortunately much less common among those who do not participate in sports. Therefore, some may argue that the principle of nonmaleficence dictates that we ban sports altogether, or at least those with a relatively high risk of sport-related concussion. It has, however, been well established that the regular exercise involved in sports participation has substantial health benefits, including a decreased risk of obesity, heart disease, stroke, sleep apnea, mental health problems, suicide, certain cancers, and all-cause mortality. In addition, participation in sports by young athletes is associated with numerous social and psychological benefits, many of which extend into adulthood, including improved self-esteem, better cardiovascular conditioning, higher academic performance, and higher career achievement. Therefore, some argue that the principle of beneficence mandates that we encourage sports participation by all patients. Finally, the principle of respect for autonomy mandates that we allow athletes to decide for themselves whether or not the benefits involved in sports participation outweigh the risks, and that we allow athletes to consider their personal beliefs, the personal benefits they derive from sports participation, and make an informed and uninfluenced opinion about whether those benefits outweigh the risks.

Some have argued that given the risks of concussion and the potential for cumulative effects of concussions in certain sports, particularly boxing and American football, the principle of nonmaleficence mandates that physicians, policymakers, and society in general ban participation by athletes in these sports, or at least pediatric athletes wishing to participate in these sports. Others argue that the principle of beneficence mandates that we should encourage all members of society participate in organized sports. While other sports would be available if football and boxing were banned, the acceptable amount of risk for given benefits varies from person to person. Furthermore, the benefits of sports vary dramatically from person to person. The principle of autonomy mandates that we inform athletes, and for pediatric athletes their parents, of the risks and benefits involved in sports and allow them to decide for themselves whether or not, given their personal beliefs and their personal circumstances, the benefits outweigh the risks and whether or not they should participate in sports.

Summary

In summary, there are four main clusters of ethical principles used to make most medical decisions: justice, nonmaleficence, beneficence, and respect for autonomy. None is absolute or universal. In many, if not most, situations, several of these principles come into conflict. The principle that holds the greatest weight varies according to the circumstances. This is common in sports, particularly when deciding whether an athlete should participate in a given sport or return to a certain sport after having sustained an injury. Given the recent concerns regarding sport-related concussion, some have called for the banning of sports that carry a relatively high risk of concussion, particularly boxing and American football, citing the principle of nonmaleficence. Others have argued that the benefits of sports participation, even in these high-risk sports, outweigh the risk of concussion and, therefore, the principle of beneficence mandates that we encourage sports participation. Still others argue that the decision to participate belongs to athletes and, for young athletes their parents, noting that the principle of respect for autonomy mandates we allow informed athletes and their families to weigh the risks against the benefits and decide for themselves.

SECTION III

Primary Documents

Heads Up, Centers for Disease Control and Prevention (CDC)

The Centers for Disease Control and Prevention developed educational materials for parents, coaches, health care providers, schools, and athletes of varying ages, designed to raise awareness regarding concussions and improve the detection and management of concussion. The website is host to videos, fact sheets, and text. It would be too much to include here, but below is a small, modified excerpt.

WHAT IS A CONCUSSION?

A concussion is a type of traumatic brain injury—or TBI—caused by a bump, blow, or jolt to the head or by a hit to the body that causes the head and brain to move rapidly back and forth. This sudden movement can cause the brain to bounce around or twist in the skull, stretching and damaging the brain cells and creating chemical changes in the brain.

CONCUSSIONS ARE SERIOUS

Medical providers may describe a concussion as a "mild" brain injury because concussions are usually not life-threatening. Even so, the effects of a concussion can be serious.

BRAIN INJURY BASICS: CONCUSSION SIGNS AND SYMPTOMS

Children and teens who show or report one or more of the signs and symptoms listed below, or simply say they just "don't feel right" after a bump, blow, or jolt to the head or body, may have a concussion or more serious brain injury.

Concussion Signs Observed

- Can't recall events *prior to* or *after* a hit or fall.
- Appears dazed or stunned.
- Forgets an instruction, is confused about an assignment or position, or is unsure of the game, score, or opponent.
- Moves clumsily.
- Answers questions slowly.
- Loses consciousness *(even briefly)*.
- Shows mood, behavior, or personality changes.

Concussion Symptoms Reported

- Headache or "pressure" in head.
- Nausea or vomiting.
- Balance problems or dizziness, or double or blurry vision.
- Bothered by light or noise.
- Feeling sluggish, hazy, foggy, or groggy.
- Confusion, or concentration or memory problems.
- Just not "feeling right," or "feeling down".

Signs and symptoms generally show up soon after the injury. However, you may not know how serious the injury is at first and some symptoms may not show up for hours or days. For example, in the first few minutes your child or teen might be a little confused or a bit dazed, but an hour later your child might not be able to remember how he or she got hurt.

You should continue to check for signs of concussion right after the injury and a few days after the injury. If your child or teen's concussion signs or symptoms get worse, you should take him or her to the emergency department right away.

Recovery from Concussion

Rest is very important after a concussion because it helps the brain heal. Your child or teen may need to limit activities while he or she is recovering from a concussion. Physical activities or activities that involve a lot of concentration, such as studying, working on the computer, or playing video games may cause concussion symptoms (such as headache or tiredness) to come back or get worse. After a concussion, physical and cognitive activities—such as concentration and learning—should be carefully watched by a medical provider. As the days go by, your child or teen can expect to slowly feel better.

Recovery Tips

Parents can help their child or teen feel better by being active in their recovery:

Rest Is Key to Help the Brain Heal

- Have your child or teen get plenty of rest. Keep a regular sleep routine, including no late nights and no sleepovers.
- Make sure your child or teen avoids high-risk/high-speed activities that could result in another bump, blow, or jolt to the head or body, such as riding a bicycle, playing sports, climbing playground equipment, and riding roller coasters. Children and teens should not return to these types of activities until their medical provider says they are well enough.
- Share information about concussion with siblings, teachers, counselors, babysitters, coaches, and others who spend time with your child or teen. This can help them understand what has happened and how to help.

Return Slowly to Activities

- When your child's or teen's medical provider says they are well enough, make sure they return to their normal activities slowly, not all at once.
- Talk with their medical provider about when your child or teen should return to school and other activities and how you can help him or her deal with any challenges during their recovery. For example, your child may need to spend less time at school, rest often, or be given more time to take tests.
- Ask your child's or teen's medical provider when he or she can safely drive a car or ride a bike.

Talk to a Medical Provider about Concerns

- Give your child or teen only medications that are approved by their medical provider.
- If your child or teen already had a medical condition at the time of their concussion (such as ADHD or chronic headaches), it may take longer for them to recover from a concussion. Anxiety and depression may also make it harder to adjust to the symptoms of a concussion.

Post-Concussive Syndrome

While most children and teens with a concussion feel better within a couple of weeks, some will have symptoms for months or longer. Talk with your children's or teens' health care provider if their concussion symptoms do not go away or if they get worse after they return to their regular activities.

If your child or teen has concussion symptoms that last weeks to months after the injury, their medical provider may talk to you about post-concussive syndrome. While rare after only one concussion, post-concussive syndrome is believed to occur most commonly in patients with a history of multiple concussions.

There are many people who can help you and your family as your child or teen recovers. You do not have to do it alone. Keep talking with your medical provider, family members, and loved ones about how your child or teen is feeling. If you do not think he or she is getting better, tell your medical provider.

RETURNING TO SCHOOL

Most kids and teens will only need help through informal, academic adjustments as they recover from a concussion. However for kids and teens with ongoing symptoms, a variety of formal support services may be available to help them during their recovery. These support services may vary widely among states and school districts. The type of support will differ based on the needs of each student. Some of these support services may include:

- Response to Intervention Protocol (RTI)
- 504 Plan
- Individualized Education Plan (IEP)

Your child or teen may feel frustrated, sad, and even angry because she or he cannot return to school right away, keep up with schoolwork, or hang out as much with their friends. Talk often with your child or teen about this and offer your support and encouragement.

RETURNING TO SPORTS AND ACTIVITIES

After a concussion, an athlete should only return to sports practices with the approval and under the supervision of their health care provider. When available, be sure to also work closely with your team's certified athletic trainer.

Below are five gradual steps that you, along with a health care provider, should follow to help safely return an athlete to play. Remember, this is a gradual process. These steps should not be completed in one day, but instead over days, weeks, or months.

5-STEP RETURN TO PLAY PROGRESSION

It is important for an athlete's parent(s) and coach(es) to watch for concussion symptoms after each day's return to play progression activity. An athlete should only move to the next step if they do not have any new symptoms at the current step. If an athlete's symptoms come back or if he or she gets new symptoms, this is a sign that the athlete is pushing too hard. The athlete should stop these activities and the athlete's medical provider should be contacted. After more rest and no concussion symptoms, the athlete can start at the previous step.

BASELINE: BACK TO SCHOOL FIRST

Athlete is back to their regular school activities, is no longer experiencing symptoms from the injury when doing normal activities, and has the green-light from their health care provider to begin the return to play process.

STEP 1: LIGHT AEROBIC ACTIVITY

Begin with light aerobic exercise only to increase an athlete's heart rate. This means about 5 to 10 minutes on an exercise bike, walking, or light jogging. No weight lifting at this point.

STEP 2: MODERATE ACTIVITY

Continue with activities to increase an athlete's heart rate with body or head movement. This includes moderate jogging, brief running, moderate-intensity stationary biking, moderate-intensity weightlifting (less time and/or less weight from their typical routine).

STEP 3: HEAVY, NON-CONTACT ACTIVITY

Add heavy non-contact physical activity, such as sprinting/running, high-intensity stationary biking, regular weightlifting routine, non-contact sport-specific drills (in 3 planes of movement).

STEP 4: PRACTICE & FULL CONTACT

Young athlete may return to practice and full contact (if appropriate for the sport) in controlled practice.

STEP 5: COMPETITION

Young athlete may return to competition.

Source: Centers for Disease Control. *Heads Up: Brain Injury Basics.* http://www.cdc.gov/headsup/basics/index.html

Nonfatal Traumatic Brain Injuries from Sports and Recreation Activities

Below is a study conducted by the Centers for Disease Control and Prevention investigating the number of nonfatal traumatic brain injuries sustained during sports and recreation that are treated in United States Emergency departments annually. Since most such injuries are not treated in emergency rooms, but rather by athletic trainers, doctors in outpatient clinics, or simply left untreated, these visits represent only a small proportion of nonfatal traumatic brain injuries that occur during sports and recreational activities. Be sure to read the accompanying editor's note to get an estimate of the overall number of injuries, including those not treated in the emergency department.

Each year in the United States, an estimated 38 million children and adolescents participate in organized sports (*1*), and approximately 170 million adults participate in some type of physical activity not related to work (*2*). The health benefits of these activities are tempered by the risk for injury, including traumatic brain injury (TBI). CDC estimates that 1.1 million persons with TBIs are treated and released from U.S. hospital emergency departments (EDs) each year, and an additional 235,000 are hospitalized for these injuries (*3*). TBIs can result in long-term, negative health effects (e.g., memory loss and behavioral changes) (*3*). To characterize sports- and recreation-related (SR-related) TBIs among patients treated in U.S. hospital EDs, CDC analyzed data from the National Electronic Injury Surveillance System—All Injury Program (NEISS-AIP) for the period 2001–2005. This report summarizes the results of that analysis, which indicated that an estimated 207,830 patients with nonfatal SR-related TBIs were treated in EDs each year during this period. The highest rates of SR-related TBI ED visits for both males and females occurred among those aged 10–14 years. Increased awareness of TBI risks, prevention strategies, and the importance of timely identification and management is essential for reducing the incidence, severity, and long-term negative health effects of this type of injury.

NEISS-AIP is operated by the U.S. Consumer Product Safety Commission (CPSC) and contains data on initial visits for all types and causes of injuries in patients treated in U.S. EDs. NEISS-AIP data are drawn from a nationally representative subsample of 66 of 100 NEISS hospitals that are selected as a stratified probability sample of those hospitals in the United States and its territories with a minimum of six beds and a 24-hour ED. NEISS-AIP provides data on approximately 500,000 injury-related and consumer-product—related ED cases each year.

For this analysis, SR-related injuries included those that occurred during organized and unorganized SR-related activities, regardless of whether they were work-related. Each case was initially classified into one of 39 mutually exclusive SR-related groups on the basis of an algorithm that considered both the consumer products involved (e.g., bicycles, swing sets, or in-line skating equipment) and the narrative description of the incident obtained from the medical record. These categories were combined for the analysis as necessary to produce stable estimates. SR-related cases were excluded if 1) the principal diagnosis was an illness, pain only, psychological harm only, contact dermatitis associated with consumer products or plants, or unknown; 2) the ED visit resulted from the adverse effects of therapeutic drugs or surgical care; or 3) the injury was violence-related, including intentional self-harm, assault, or legal intervention. Because not all deaths are counted by NEISS-AIP, persons who were dead on arrival or who died in the ED also were excluded. SR-related injury cases were then classified as TBI cases if the primary body part injured was the head and the principal diagnosis was within the categories of concussion or internal organ injury.

Each case was assigned a sample weight on the basis of the inverse probability of selection; these weights were added to provide national estimates of SR-related injuries. Estimates were based on weighted data for 347,597 ED visits for SR-related injuries (of which 21,876 were for TBI) during 2001–2005. Confidence intervals were calculated using a direct variance estimation procedure that accounted for the sample weights and complex sample design (4). Rates were calculated using averaged 2001–2005 U.S. Census bridged-race population estimates (5).

During 2001–2005, an estimated 207,830 patients with SR-related TBIs were treated in U.S. hospital EDs each year, accounting for 5.1% of all SR-related ED visits (Table III.1). Overall, males accounted for approximately 70.5% of SR-related TBI ED visits. The highest rates of SR-related TBI ED visits for both males and females occurred among those aged 10–14 years, followed by those aged 15–19 years (Figure III.1). Activities associated with the greatest number of TBI-related ED visits included bicycling, football, playground activities, basketball, and riding all-terrain vehicles (ATVs). Activities for which TBI accounted for greater than 7.5% of ED visits for that activity included horseback riding (11.7%), ice skating (10.4%), riding ATVs (8.4%), tobogganing/sledding

(8.3%), and bicycling (7.7%). Each year, an estimated 21,311 SR-related TBI ED visits occurred that involved patients who were either subsequently hospitalized or transferred to another facility for additional care (Table III.2). Approximately 10.3% of patients with SR-related TBIs were hospitalized or transferred, compared with 3.1% of patients with SR-related injuries overall. Activities associated with the greatest proportion of TBI-related ED visits requiring either hospitalization or transfer included riding ATVs (30.2%), riding mopeds/minibikes/dirt bikes (21.9%), bicycling (15.6%), golfing (13.6%), and riding scooters (10.5%).

During 2001–2005, children aged 5–18 years accounted for an estimated 2.4 million (59.7%) SR-related ED visits, of which approximately 134,959 (5.6%) were categorized as TBI-related (Table III.1). Approximately 17.9% of SR-related hospitalizations in this age group were attributed to TBIs (Table III.2). Activities associated with the greatest number of TBI-related ED visits in this age group included bicycling, football, basketball, playground activities, and soccer. For all ages, activities for which TBI accounted for the greatest proportion of ED visits for that activity and the activities associated with the greatest number of TBI-related ED visits resulting in hospitalization were similar.

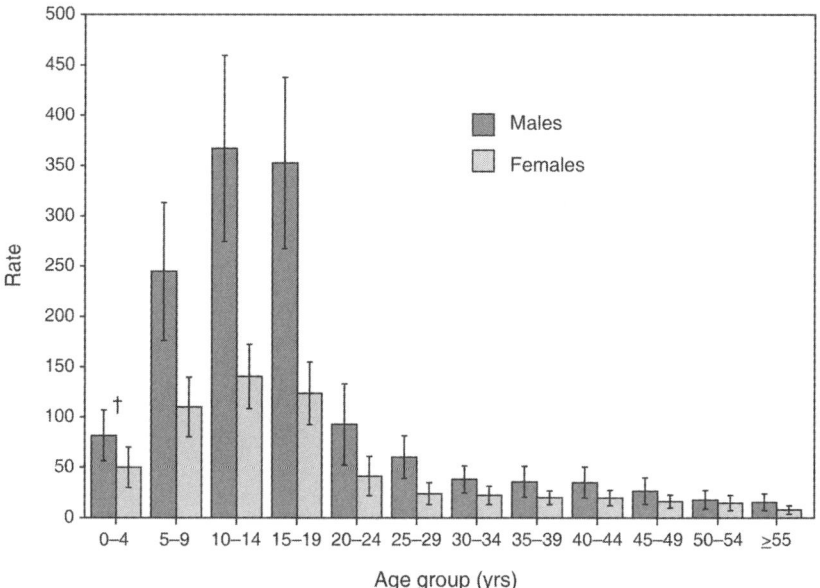

* Per 100,000 population.
† 95% confidence interval.

Figure 1 Estimated annual rate* of nonfatal, sports- and recreation-related traumatic brain injuries treated in emergency departments, by age group and sex—National Electronic Injury Surveillance System-All Injury Program, United States, 2001–2005

TABLE III.1 Estimated annual number of emergency department (ED) visits for all nonfatal injuries and nonfatal traumatic brain injuries (TBIs) related to sports and recreation activities, for all ages and for ages 5–18 years, by activity—National Electronic Injury Surveillance System-All Injury Program, United States, 2001–2005

Activity	All ages					Ages 5–18 yrs						
	All injuries		TBIs			All injuries		TBIs				
	No.*	(95% CI†)	No.	(95% CI)	% of all injuries§	No.	(95% CI)	No.	(95% CI)	% of all injuries	% of all injuries in age group¶	% of TBIs in age group**
Bicycle	524,692	(434,500–614,883)	40,424	(25,293–55,555)	7.7	309,752	(263,097–356,407)	23,405	(16,860–29,950)	7.6	59.0	57.9
Football	398,369	(349,189–447,550)	22,689	(18,102–27,276)	5.7	320,542	(277,524–363,560)	20,293	(16,255–24,332)	6.3	80.5	89.4
Playground	226,091	(186,257–265,925)	16,130	(11,004–21,256)	7.1	160,621	(133,056–188,186)	10,414	(7,185–13,644)	6.5	71.0	64.6
Basketball	603,239	(528,121–678,357)	14,680	(10,782–18,579)	2.4	380,245	(328,566–431,924)	11,506	(8,528–14,485)	3.0	63.0	78.4
All-terrain vehicle	132,702	(101,439–163,964)	11,199	(5,856–16,542)	8.4	53,447	(40,562–66,332)	5,220	(2,462–7,979)	9.8	40.3	46.6
Baseball	163,215	(136,676–189,755)	10,103	(7,414–12,792)	6.2	113,649	(93,833–133,465)	7,433	(5,440–9,426)	6.5	69.6	73.6
Soccer	169,373	(120,915–217,830)	9,371	(5,753–12,989)	5.5	122,731	(87,045–158,417)	7,667	(4,747–10,588)	6.2	72.5	81.8
Horseback riding	74,096	(55,856–92,336)	8,650	(4,496–12,803)	11.7	20,903	(15,972–25,834)	2,648	(1,593–3,704)	12.7	28.2	30.6
Swimming/diving	99,514	(74,848–124,179)	5,878	(3,398–8,357)	5.9	52,684	(41,271–64,098)	3,846	(2,325–5,367)	7.3	52.9	65.4
Skateboard	109,550	(72,553–146,546)	5,292	(3,124–7,460)	4.8	86,765	(60,612–112,918)	4,408	(2,561–6,255)	5.1	79.2	83.3
Hockey††	70,548	(34,650–106,445)	5,194	(2,239–8,149)	7.4	45,127	(20,554–69,700)	4,111§§	(1,523–6,699)	9.1§§	64.0	79.1§§
Moped/minibike/dirt bike¶¶	71,987	(55,405–88,569)	4,736	(3,023–6,449)	6.6	33,868	(25,092–42,643)	2,523	(1,677–3,370)	7.5	47.0	53.3
Softball	108,014	(87,021–129,007)	4,277	(2,967–5,588)	4.0	45,153	(35,611–54,695)	1,797	(1,171–2,423)	4.0	41.8	42.0
Exercise	230,966	(193,241–268,691)	4,163	(2,368–5,958)	1.8	62,226	(52,865–71,587)	1,469	(863–2,076)	2.4	26.9	35.3
Miscellaneous ball games***	89,469	(71,798–107,140)	3,814	(2,211–5,416)	4.3	59,338	(46,559–72,116)	2,470	(1,634–3,306)	4.2	66.3	64.8
Combative†††	77,088	(62,232–91,944)	3,682	(2,537–4,827)	4.8	46,488	(36,219–56,757)	2,456	(1,627–3,284)	5.3	60.3	66.7
Scooter	67,197	(53,340–81,054)	3,534	(2,558–4,511)	5.3	52,355	(42,058–62,652)	2,790	(2,061–3,518)	5.3	77.9	78.9
Gymnastics§§§	93,603	(77,169–110,037)	2,951	(2,038–3,864)	3.2	64,507	(51,567–77,447)	2,339	(1,579–3,100)	3.6	68.9	79.3
Toboggan/sled	32,279	(20,161–44,397)	2,687	(1,411–3,964)	8.3	21,292	(13,340–29,245)	1,873	(1,011–2,736)	8.8	66.0	69.7
Golf¶¶¶	40,578	(30,313–50,843)	2,687	(1,783–3,591)	6.6	13,058	(10,092–16,023)	1,125	(681–1,569)	8.6	32.2	41.9
Skating, ice	23,214	(15,810–30,618)	2,411	(1,546–3,275)	10.4	14,387	(9,666–19,108)	1,545	(909–2,181)	10.7	62.0	64.1
Trampoline	93,389	(73,452–113,325)	2,131	(1,382–2,881)	2.3	73,029	(57,219–88,839)	1,545	(1,013–2,078)	2.1	78.2	72.5
Skating, in-line	46,665	(32,989–60,342)	1,610	(982–2,238)	3.5	33,109	(23,692–42,525)	1,142	(742–1,542)	3.4	70.9	70.9

Activity							
Skating, other****	53,795 (41,434–66,156)	2.7	36,609 (28,152–45,066)	1,087 (749–1,425)	3.0	68.1	74.6
Amusement attractions†††	21,273 (15,270–27,275)	6.5	10,947 (7,698–14,196)	859 (467–1,250)	7.8	51.5	61.7
Go-cart	16,951 (13,235–20,667)	7.3	11,336 (8,835–13,838)	872 (521–1,223)	7.7	66.9	70.2
Volleyball	56,620 (43,298–69,942)	2.1	31,694 (24,700–38,689)	904 (581–1,227)	2.9	56.0	77.2
Racquet sports§§§§	28,268 (20,428–36,108)	2.6	8,299 (6,408–10,191)	198§§ (71–325)	2.4§§	29.4	27.4§§
Bowling	18,978 (14,628–23,329)	2.1	4,863 (3,665–6,061)	93§§ (24–163)	1.9§§	25.6	23.7§§
Track and field	17,025 (13,528–20,523)	1.8	15,391 (12,179–18,602)	275 (116–435)	1.8	90.4	90.2
Other specified	287,595 (181,598–393,593)	4.5	111,552 (66,868–156,236)	6,643§§ (2,137–11,149)	6.0§§	38.8	51.7§§
Total	**4,046,344 (3,443,054–4,649,635)**	**5.1**	**2,415,968 (2,047,424–2,784,512)**	**134,959 (102,530–167,388)**	**5.6**	**59.7**	**64.9**

* Estimates might not sum to totals because of rounding.

† Confidence interval.

§ Percentage of all injuries attributed to TBI = (number of TBI-related ED visits for activity/total number of ED visits for activity) × 100.

¶ Percentage of all injuries in age group = (number of sports- and recreation-related [SR-related] ED visits for activity in persons aged 5–18 years/number of SR-related ED visits for activity in persons of all ages) × 100.

** Percentage of TBIs in age group = (number of SR-related TBI ED visits for activity in persons aged 5–18 years/number of SR-related TBI ED visits for activity in persons of all ages) × 100.

†† Includes ice hockey, field hockey, roller hockey, and street hockey.

§§ Estimate might be unstable because the coefficient of variation is >30%.

¶¶ Includes other two-wheeled, powered off-road vehicles and dune buggies.

*** Includes lacrosse, rugby, handball, and tetherball.

††† Includes boxing, wrestling, martial arts, and fencing.

§§§ Includes cheerleading and dancing.

¶¶¶ Includes injuries related to golf carts.

**** Includes roller skating.

†††† Includes rides and water slides (not swimming pool slides).

§§§§ Includes tennis, badminton, and squash.

¶¶¶¶ Includes water skiing, surfing, personal watercraft, snow skiing, snowmobile, snowboarding, camping, fishing, archery, darts, table tennis, nonpowder/BB guns, and billiards.

TABLE III.2 Estimated annual number of hospitalizations* for all nonfatal injuries and nonfatal traumatic brain injuries (TBIs) related to sports and recreation activities, for all ages and for ages 5–18 years, by selected activity—National Electronic Injury Surveillance System-All Injury Program, United States, 2001–2005

Activity	All ages						Ages 5–18 years					
	All injuries		TBIs		% of all injury hospitalizations¶	% resulting in hospitalization**	All injuries		TBIs		% of all injury resulting in hospitalizations	
	No.†	(95% CI§)	No.	(95% CI)			No.	(95% CI)	No.	(95% CI)		
Bicycle	25,062	(17,858–32,267)	6,296	(3,636–8,957)	25.1	15.6	11,396	(8,958–13,835)	3,026	(1,993–4,059)	26.6	12.9
All-terrain vehicle	16,503	(10,195–22,810)	3,383	(1,649–5,117)	20.5	30.2	6,413	(3,897–8,929)	1,622	(698–2,545)	25.3	31.1
Moped/minibike/dirt bike††	6,095	(3,848–8,341)	1,039	(442–1,636)	17.0	21.9	2,653	(1,683–3,623)	517	(233–801)	19.5	20.5
Football	6,809	(5,588–8,030)	891	(633–1,148)	13.1	3.9	5,639	(4,590–6,688)	775	(521–1,029)	13.7	3.8
Baseball/softball	3,759	(2,895–4,623)	811	(491–1,130)	21.6	5.6	1,926	(1,481–2,371)	419	(198–640)	21.8	4.5
Playground	9,669	(7,714–11,624)	529	(332–727)	5.5	3.3	7,398	(5,727–9,069)	349	(200–497)	4.7	3.3
Basketball	4,816	(4,057–5,575)	465	(274–656)	9.7	3.2	2,674	(2,110–3,238)	365	(218–513)	13.6	3.2
Skateboard	3,068	(1,700–4,437)	432	(216–647)	14.1	8.2	2,304	(1,389–3,219)	350	(170–529)	15.2	7.9
Scooter	2,011	(1,586–2,437)	372	(191–552)	18.5	10.5	1,429	(1,090–1,769)	329	(154–504)	23.0	11.8
Golf§§	1,586	(1,016–2,156)	366	(159–573)	23.1	13.6	504	(299–708)	178	(87–269)	35.3	15.8
Swimming/diving	3,915	(2,380–5,449)	352	(155–549)	9.0	6.0	1,304	(820–1,789)	198	(81–315)	15.2	5.1
Skating¶¶	2,946	(2,148–3,745)	263	(126–399)	8.9	4.8	1,571	(1,114–2,029)	153	(63–243)	9.7	4.0
Soccer	2,653	(1,625–3,681)	198	(84–312)	7.5	2.1	1,602	(999–2,206)	161	(66–256)	10.0	2.1
Other specified***	37,790	(27,470–48,110)	5,916	(3,264–8,567)	15.7	11.5	13,557	(10,359–16,755)	2,351	(1,340–3,361)	17.3	8.2
Total	**126,683**	**(97,146–156,220)**	**21,311**	**(13,258–29,364)**	**16.8**	**10.3**	**60,372**	**(49,416–71,329)**	**10,790**	**(7,461–14,120)**	**17.9**	**8.0**

* Includes those for patients hospitalized and those for patients transferred to another facility for additional care.

† Estimates might not sum to totals because of rounding.

§ Confidence interval.

¶ Percentage of all hospitalizations attributed to TBI = (number of TBI hospitalizations for activity/number of all hospitalizations for activity) × 100.

** Percentage of TBIs resulting in hospitalization = (number of TBI hospitalizations for activity/number of TBI-related emergency department visits for activity).

†† Includes other two-wheeled, powered off-road vehicles and dune buggies.

§§ Includes injuries related to golf carts.

¶¶ Includes ice, in-line, and roller skating.

*** Includes trampoline, toboggan/sled, go-cart, gymnastics, bowling, hockey, racquet sports, volleyball, miscellaneous ball games, track/field, combative, exercise, amusement attractions, water skiing, surfing, personal watercraft, snow skiing, snowmobile, snowboarding, camping, fishing, archery, darts, table tennis, nonpowder/BB guns, and billiards.

Editorial Note

The findings in this report indicate that an estimated 207,830 patients with SR-related TBIs were treated in U.S. EDs each year during 2001–2005. TBIs can occur during any of these SR-related activities, at any age, and among persons of either sex. Previous research has demonstrated that the majority of TBIs are categorized initially as mild on the basis of signs and symptoms; however, even mild TBI can affect a person's ability to return to school or work and can result in long-term cognitive or other problems (3). Repeated or more severe TBIs can result in physical, cognitive, behavioral, or emotional problems (6).

A previous national estimate of 300,000 SR-related TBIs included only those TBIs involving loss of consciousness (7). However, two studies have reported that only 8%–19% of SR-related TBIs involve loss of consciousness (8,9). An extrapolation based on these parameters suggests that 1.6–3.8 million SR-related TBIs occur each year, including those not treated by a health-care provider (3). Based on this estimate and the results of the analysis described in this report, an estimated 5.5%–13.0% of SR-related TBIs might result in hospital ED visits each year. Data on ED visits provide the most available national estimates for tracking this public health problem; however, the actual burden is underrepresented by use of these data. Although the information derived from NEISS-AIP in this report reflects only a limited portion of all SR-related TBIs (i.e., those resulting in ED visits), the information is useful because it enables the classification of types of SR-related activities. Other injury classification systems (e.g., *International Classification of Diseases, Ninth Revision, Clinical Modification*) do not enable coding of the specific SR-related activity involved at the time of injury.

The findings in this report indicate that persons aged 5–18 years account for an estimated 60% of ED visits for SR-related injuries and 65% of ED visits for SR-related TBIs. Persons in this age group are at increased risk for concussion during SR-related activities and for long-term sequelae, delayed recovery, and cumulative consequences of multiple TBIs (e.g., increased severity of future TBIs and increased risk for depression and dementia) (3,10). Therefore, prevention measures should be targeted to this age group.

To improve diagnosis and management of mild TBIs, including concussions, CDC has developed a tool kit for physicians entitled "Heads Up: Brain Injury in Your Practice." In addition, CDC recently released a new tool kit, "Heads Up: Concussion in Youth Sports," to accompany an existing tool kit, "Heads Up: Concussion in High School Sports." This new tool kit was developed to help youth sports coaches and administrators, parents, and athletes better understand how to prevent, recognize, and respond to concussion among young athletes. The tool kit contains 1) fact sheets for coaches, parents, and athletes; 2) a clipboard, magnet, and poster containing facts on concussion; and 3) a quiz for coaches, athletes, and parents to test their knowledge about concussion.

Key components of TBI prevention in SR-related activities include 1) using protective equipment appropriate for the sport or activity (e.g., a helmet) that fits properly and is worn correctly and consistently, 2) following all appropriate safety policies, and 3) following the rules of the sport. In addition, all players, parents, and coaches should be aware of the signs and symptoms of TBIs, including concussion, and take appropriate action when such an injury is suspected. Additional information about the "Heads Up: Concussion in Youth Sports" tool kit (including information about ordering the kit free of charge) is available at http://www.cdc .gov/concussioninyouthsports.

The findings in this report are subject to at least six limitations. First, injury rates for specific SR-related activities could not be calculated because of the lack of national data regarding the number of persons participating in SR-related activities. Therefore, these estimates cannot be used to calculate the risks for TBI associated with any particular sport or activity. Second, NEISS-AIP includes only injuries resulting in visits to hospital EDs; many persons with TBIs do not seek care in EDs. Third, because NEISS-AIP includes only the principal diagnosis and primary body part noted during the initial injury visit, some cases for which TBI was a secondary diagnosis might have been missed. Fourth, NEISS-AIP narrative descriptions do not provide detailed information about injury circumstances (e.g., whether the activity was organized, whether the injury occurred during training or competition, or whether protective equipment was used). Fifth, trends by year could not be calculated because small numbers would have resulted in unstable estimates. Finally, NEISS-AIP is designed to provide national estimates but not state or local estimates.

These estimates highlight the need to improve the recognition, management, and prevention of SR-related TBIs and to better track the actual extent of this health problem. Additional information and resources on TBI, including all tool kits, are available at http://www.cdc.gov/ncipc/tbi/tbi.htm.

REFERENCES

1. National Council on Youth Sports. Report on trends and participation in youth sports. Stuart, FL: National Council on Youth Sports; 2001. Available at http://www.ncys.org/pdf/marketresearch.pdf.
2. CDC. 2006 Behavioral Risk Factor Surveillance System. Available at http:// apps.nccd.cdc.gov/brfss/display.asp?cat=ex&yr=2006&qkey=4347&state=ub.
3. Langlois JA, Rutland-Brown W, Wald MM. The epidemiology and impact of traumatic brain injury. J Head Trauma Rehabil 2006;21: 375–8.
4. US Consumer Product Safety Commission. NEISS All Injury Program: sample design and implementation. Schroeder T, Ault K, preparers. Washington, DC: US Consumer Product Safety Commission, 2001.
5. CDC. U.S. census populations with bridged race categories. Hyattsville, MD: US Department of Health and Human Services, CDC; 2006. Available at http://www.cdc.gov/nchs/about/major/dvs/popbridge/popbridge.htm.
6. National Institutes of Health. Rehabilitation of persons with traumatic brain injury: NIH consensus statement. Bethesda, MD: National Institutes of Health; 1998. Available at http://consensus.nih.gov/1998/1998traumaticbrain injury109html.htm.

7. Thurman DJ, Branche CM, Sniezek JE. The epidemiology of sports-related traumatic brain injuries in the United States: recent developments. J Head Trauma Rehabil 1998;13: 1–8.

8. Schultz MR, Marshall SW, Mueller FO, et al. Incidence and risk factors for concussion in high school athletes, North Carolina, 1996–1999. Am J Epidemiol 2004;160:937–44.

9. Collins MW, Iverson GL, Lovell MR, McKeag DB, Norwig J, Maroon J. On-field predictors of neuropsychological and symptom deficit following sports-related concussion. Clin J Sport Med 2003; 13:222–9.

10. Buzzini SR, Guskiewicz KM. Sport-related concussion in the young athlete. Curr Opin Pediatr 2006;18:376–82.

Source: J. Gilchrist, K. E. Thomas, M. Wald, and J. Langlois. "Nonfatal Traumatic Brain Injuries from Sports and Recreation Activities—United States, 2001–2005." *Morbidity and Mortality Weekly Report* 2007; 56(29): 733–737.

Concussions and the Marketing of Sports Equipment: Hearing before Congress, October 19, 2011

Research is a tricky thing. Due to the limitations of statistics and the probability of random occurrences, you can find a research article that shows just about anything. That is why in medicine and science, we rarely base our decisions on a single research project, but rather assess the overall body of studies on a given topic when drawing conclusions. Lately, some manufacturers of sports equipment have been advertising to athletes and parents that their equipment can prevent concussions. While this may be an effective marketing tool, the evidence supporting such claims is scant. Congress held a hearing to address the concern that such advertising was misleading to consumers, calling in experts to interpret the overall body of evidence. Some selections from the transcript from that hearing are below.

The Committee met, pursuant to notice, at 2:34 p.m., in room SR-253, Russell Senate Office Building, Hon. John D. Rockefeller IV, Chairman of the Committee, presiding . . .

    . . . every afternoon at the end of the school day, millions of our children head to playing fields, gymnasiums, or hockey rinks to participate in team sports. I should have said soccer fields, too. Playing sports doesn't just make our kids stronger and healthier. It also teaches them important values. They learn about hard work, about leadership, about living with pain and going through it, about working together for a common goal.

    The camaraderie that comes out of sports units is wonderful to see. It is real, and it lasts forever. Most of our young athletes will not end up playing sports at the collegiate or professional level, but we hope they will all carry the positive lessons they have learned on the playing fields with them throughout life, and they will.

So our hearing today is about the head injuries that tens of thousands of these athletes sustain every year while playing the sports they love. Many of us are reluctant to talk about the risks involved in playing sports because we know what a positive role that sports play in our communities.

On the other hand, the last thing we can do here is not talk about this problem of concussions and gear and all the rest of it. I mean, America has to have this conversation, and there will be many, many hearings on it, I know.

In fact, more of our children should be playing sports, not fewer. Too many kids are spending their afternoons in front of computer or televisions screens, instead of on the sports field. And that is said every day by everybody who is involved in healthcare. I am going to give you a couple of pathetic figures.

According to the latest data compiled by the Centers for Disease Control, only 17 percent of American high school students get an hour of daily physical activity, which is our current health guidelines. They say that, that you need to have that to stay healthy—only 17 percent. One-third of our children are now overweight or obese, which makes it more likely that they will suffer from chronic health conditions, such as heart disease or diabetes, things which will plague them for the rest of their lives as, indeed, what we will be talking about today could do to some.

But the risks involved in playing sports are also very, very real. And by now, we have all heard about the National Football League players who are struggling with serious mental and physical health problems because they sustained repeated mild traumatic brain injuries, which is what concussions are called, I guess, medically, during their playing years. And it is very, very sad.

I mean, I have seen a number of these players, people that I had worshipped growing up, in wheelchairs. Who was the guy that played—he was a cornerback for the Raiders? The greatest interceptor of all time, Woody—come on, give me——

No. No. Doesn't matter. Doesn't matter.

[Laughter.]

The Chairman. But I mean, it was awful. I was at an event with him, and he was seated in a wheelchair, and he couldn't even pull his head up. And I leaned down and whispered in his ear. I think I kissed him, too. I am not sure. But it was having seen from this to that and who knows, especially this was 8 years ago. Nobody was talking about it.

We now understand, however, that this is not an injury only NFL players can suffer. According to research conducted at the Nationwide Children's Hospital in Columbus, Ohio, more than 70,000 high school football players sustain concussions every single year.

And it is not just a football problem. One of our witnesses today, Alexis Ball, will talk about the concussions she suffered while playing soccer in high school and college. According to Nationwide Children's Hospital, more than 10,000 high school girl soccer players sustain concussions each year.

So what we are going to do is we are going to hear from Ms. Ball and our other witnesses today, who I should name. Dr. Jeffrey Kutcher. Jeffrey, you are not in my opening script. So I have to do this, and you forgive me. Associate Professor, Department of Neurology, University of Michigan; Director, Michigan NeuroSport. And Dr. Ann McKee, Professor of Neurology and Pathology at Boston University and Director of Neuropathology Core, BU Alzheimer's Disease Center. I guess that is Boston University's. And Mr. Mike Oliver, who is Executive Director of the National Operating Committee on Standards for Athletic Equipment.

We welcome all of you, and I will just close right there and ask if the Chairman of the Subcommittee would wish to say something because he has been just terrific on this subject and also the Ranking Member.

Go ahead.

STATEMENT OF HON. JOHN BOOZMAN, U.S. SENATOR FROM ARKANSAS

Senator Boozman. Well, thank you, Mr. Chairman, again for us holding this very important hearing this afternoon.

As a former player, it is certainly something that I am interested in. But also there are so many moms and dads and coaches and players all across the country that also are very interested and probably should be more interested than what they realize. And I think that is the great thing about having this hearing is to try and get that information out and really discuss a potential very serious problem. Not a potential very serious problem, a very serious problem, period.

Sports play a vital role in development of young men and women. They help build youth social relationships and learn to work as a team while keeping them physically active and healthy and having fun. According to the National High School Sports-Related Injury Surveillance Study, participation in high school sports has almost doubled in the last 30 years.

This is fantastic news, and I think it is important for us to highlight the benefits of playing sports. However, participation in athletics does carry with it significant risk of injury. Just last week, there was news of a tragic death of a 16-year-old high school football player who died after sustaining a head injury during a game.

It is important that everyone—coaches, parents, physicians, and the athletes themselves—understand those risks and be able to identify injuries when they occur. Concussions especially have the potential for severe injury, and multiple concussions can cause significant repercussions later in life, as we are going to hear about today.

Especially with many recent media reports of high-profile incidents in the NFL, we often associate football with concussions. As I am well aware and as Mr. Threet will mention in his testimony, concussions are a risk with playing football, but players in many sports run the risk of sustaining concussion, as we will hear from Ms. Ball in her story about playing soccer.

It is imperative for coaches and parents involved in all sports to be aware of the dangers associated with concussions, know how to recognize the signs and symptoms and what to do if a player suffers a concussion. I look forward to hearing from Dr. Kutcher and Dr. McKee about the research to further the knowledge that we have about concussions, but many questions remain as to the causes and effects of concussions. I am very interested in hearing from the experts on what is known and where we can go from here.

As we will also discuss, there is a wide variety of athletic equipment on the market that claim to use concussion-reducing or concussion-preventing technology. Parents want to keep their children protected, but navigating the many products and claims in the marketplace, especially online, can be overwhelming. It can be easy to read that something offers the best maximum security protection and assume that their child will be safe from injury. That is simply not true.

Some products may offer better protection than others, but we need to explore what resources exist to help parents and coaches know what level of safety a product will actually provide. I also do not know how the average parent or coach can be confident that the equipment they purchase genuinely offers a greater safety benefit or if its advertisement contains misleading or deceptive claims. I hope our witnesses today will be able to help me answer this question.

Along with knowing the safety benefits and limitations of sports equipment, parents and coaches need to educate themselves on what to look for in the event that an athlete has a potential concussion. There are a number of different materials available for this purpose. Perhaps the most well-known education effort is the "Heads Up" initiative, led by the CDC in partnership with dozens of professional organizations and individuals.

Individual associations, like USA Football, also have their own education campaigns for coaches, how to teach proper execution of plays and tackles so athletes are in as little danger as possible. However, education campaigns must be effective in order to effect change. I am interested to learn if there is data that shows whether these efforts are reaching a wide enough audience and promoting awareness sufficiently.

Mr. Chairman, I know today's hearing will draw attention to this important safety issue. Parents, coaches, and athletes must have the resources available to them to understand the severity of concussions and how to react when one occurs. As I said earlier, the benefits from participating in sports are many, and I hope that the potential for injury does not prevent anyone from playing.

Mr. Chairman, again, I thank you for calling this very important hearing and look forward to hearing from our witnesses. I ask unanimous consent that a statement from the Sporting Goods Manufacturers Association and USA Football be in the record.

The Chairman. It is so done.

Senator Boozman. And with that, I yield back.

The Chairman. I thank the Senator and call upon Senator Udall, who has been huge in putting together all of this.

STATEMENT OF HON. TOM UDALL, U.S. SENATOR FROM NEW MEXICO

Senator Udall. Thank you, Chairman Rockefeller, and thank you for that nice comment.

And I very much appreciate you holding this hearing today. I would like to say a few words and ask that my full statement be put in the record. And Mr. Chairman, I greatly appreciate your efforts to promote brain research and, as Chairman of this Subcommittee, your close attention to consumer protection issues.

Concussions used to be dismissed as simply "dings" or "bell-ringers." We know now that a concussion is a form of traumatic brain injury that should be taken seriously. According to a recent Centers for Disease Control report, emergency room visits for sports and recreation-related traumatic brain injuries increased by 60 percent among children and adolescents over the last decade.

The CDC attributes this rise to greater concussion awareness, which is a good thing. Now that athletes, coaches, and parents have a better understanding of concussions, some sports equipment makers appear to be taking advantage. There are a number of so-called "anti-concussion" and "concussion-reducing" devices on the market.

While we should encourage any innovation to protect young athletes, we need to make sure that advertisers play by the rules. Expert witnesses today can shed some light on "anti-concussion" claims used by some sports equipment manufacturers.

Although we now know more about the dangers of concussions, we shouldn't forget how important sports and physical activity is for children. The CDC estimates that only 18 percent of American high school students participate in at least 1 hour of physical activity a day. That is the amount recommended by the Department of Health and Human Services.

Among high school students in New Mexico, only 23 percent are getting it. This could lead to negative health consequences that last a lifetime. So we need to encourage kids to play sports, to exercise, and to be more physically active. Injury is always a risk, but the benefits far outweigh the dangers. And as we learn more about the dangers of concussions for young athletes, we can take steps to make sure that they are played more safely.

I want to thank all the witnesses for being here and testifying today. I especially want to recognize Ms. Alexis Ball, who traveled from Albuquerque to share her experience with sports concussions.

In reviewing Dr. McKee's testimony, I find it especially poignant that she discusses Dave Duerson, a former NFL player who tragically took his own life earlier this year. In 2007, he testified before this committee. According to news reports, Duerson informed his family that he wanted his brain to be studied. He hoped people could learn more about the effect of brain trauma so kids could play football more safely in the future.

In keeping with this sentiment, I hope that this hearing today will advance the goal of making sports safer for our children.

With that, Chairman Rockefeller, thank you very much, and thanks for being here and the Ranking Member for being here. Appreciate it.

The Chairman. That is a pretty powerful statement.

Senator Udall. Thank you.

[The prepared statement of Senator Udall follows:]

PREPARED STATEMENT OF THE HON. TOM UDALL, U.S. SENATOR FROM NEW MEXICO

Concussions used to be dismissed as simply "dings" or "bell ringers." Today we know that a concussion is a form of traumatic brain injury that should be taken seriously. For young people between 15 and 24 years old, playing sports is the second-leading cause of traumatic brain injury—second only to motor vehicle crashes.

According to a recent Centers for Disease Control and Prevention (CDC) report, Nonfatal Traumatic Brain Injuries Related to Sports and Recreation Activities Among Persons Aged >19 Years—United States, 2001–2009, emergency room visits for sports and recreation-related traumatic brain injuries increased by 60 percent among children and adolescents over the last decade. The CDC attributes this rise to greater concussion awareness, which is actually a good thing.

Now that athletes, coaches, and parents have a better understanding of concussions, some sports equipment makers appear to be taking advantage of their new concerns about safety. There are a number of so-called "anti-concussion" and "concussion reducing" devices on the market—from helmets and headbands to mouth guards, and even dietary supplements. While we should encourage any innovation to protect young athletes, we need to make sure that advertisers play by the rules. Claims they make about the safety of their equipment should be truthful and not misleading. Expert witnesses today can shed light on some of these concussions-related claims, and I look forward to hearing their testimony.

Earlier this year, I asked the Federal Trade Commission (FTC) to investigate some of the safety claims used to sell football helmets. Given the seriousness of concussion risk and the potential for real injury to children, the FTC should have the ability to impose civil penalties, at the agency's discretion, for any violation of the FTC Act that involves the use of false injury prevention claims to sell children's sports gear.

I also introduced legislation. This bill, the Children's Sports Athletic Equipment Safety Act, would allow the FTC to impose civil penalties for using false injury prevention claims to sell any kind of children's sports equipment. Again, under my bill the use of this enforcement power would be at the agency's discretion. It would also require improvements to the current voluntary safety standard for football helmets. I am pleased to be working on this important legislation in a bipartisan manner with Representatives Bill Pascrell and Todd Russell Platts, the Co-Chairs of the Congressional Brain Injury Task Force. I also want to thank fellow Commerce Committee member Sen. Lautenberg for his support and co-sponsorship of the legislation.

I believe it is important to share with my Commerce committee colleagues some of the potentially misleading advertising that is used to market so-called "anti-concussion" and "concussion reducing" sports gear for children's use.

My January 4, 2011 letter to FTC Chairman Jon Leibowitz cited several troubling advertisements for youth football helmets in particular. For example, one troubling claim comes from Riddell, the leading helmet-maker in the country. Riddell continues to use a concussion reduction claim that appears to be deceptive, misleading, and unsubstantiated.

The CEO of Riddell, Dan Arment, told the House Committee on the Judiciary at a January 4, 2010 hearing on "Legal Issues Relating to Football Head Injuries" that:

> "We have independent, peer-reviewed, published research in the medical journal Neurosurgery, February of 2006, showing that the Revolution [helmet] reduces the risks of concussions by 31 percent when compared to traditional helmets . . . Today, over one million high school, college, and professional players have made the switch from traditional helmets to the Revolution family of helmets." (See also "House Judiciary Committee hearing—Dan Arment opening statement." Video recording. Available at http://www.youtube.com/watch?feature=player_embedded&v=v1gmwk2nqi4 accessed Oct. 19, 2011)

Riddell bases this claim on a single study of high school football players using brand new Riddell Revolution helmets compared with players wearing used and reconditioned helmets of unknown condition. Scientists who commented on the article cautioned against drawing broad conclusions from a single study that compared the performance of new helmets with used headgear of unknown condition and that examined just 136 high school players who experienced concussions.

Nevertheless, Riddell launched a media campaign featuring the claim from the 2006 study that, according to its "Riddell Revolution UPMC Media Campaign Highlights" video news release, created "over 60 million media impressions, nearly 150 television placements, over 100 newspaper clips, over 250 on-line placements, [and] 6 live sports radio interviews." (See http://www.riddell.com/pressreleases_upmcstudy/, accessed Jan. 6, 2011.)

Several helmet and sports safety experts have criticized Riddell's use of this concussion prevention claim to sell Revolution type helmets. In his 2007 book, Head Games: Football's Concussion Crisis from the NFL to Youth Leagues, Chris Nowinski notes that:

> "As it is well established that rotational forces have a major role in football concussions, and that football helmets do little to reduce those forces, we could skip the discussion of the benefits of the newest football helmets, the Riddell 'Revolution' and the Schutt 'DNA.' If they make any difference it all, it would be minor. But . . . both these companies are spending a lot of money to get you to buy these newer and more expensive helmets. You deserve to know what's really going on."

In his book, Nowinski also quotes Dr. Robert Cantu, a board member of the National Operating Committee on Standards for Athletic Equipment (NOCSAE), who told him that:

"The theory behind the [Riddell] 'Revolution' is that if you build a helmet that's a little bit bigger, especially in the temple area, and padded more thickly, then you'll reduce force more than you would if you had thinner padding and not so big an outer shell. That theory is good for blows that go right to the temple, but that's it."

NOCSAE's technical director, Dave Halstead, told the New York Times in an October 27, 2007 story titled "Studies for Competing Design Called Into Question" that ". . . the [Riddell] Revolution is a good Helmet . . . But I have problems with that particular [2006 Neurosurgery] study. The helmet is not shown to do what they say it does." In another October 21, 2010 New York Times article titled "As Injuries Rise, Scant Oversight of Helmet Safety," Halstead bluntly told reporter Alan Schwarz that ". . . I don't believe that 31 percent [reduction in concussion risk claim] for a Yankee minute." These public statements from one author of the 2006 study and other helmet safety experts call into question whether there is competent and reliable scientific evidence to substantiate Riddell's marketing claim.

Moreover, Riddell advertisements cited in my letter to the FTC do not disclose that the company provided a grant to underwrite the 2006 Neurosurgery study. Nor do they disclose that Riddell's vice president of research and development, Thad Ide, was one of the study authors. An official Neurosurgery commenter highlighted the authors' conflicts of interest and stated that the study's conclusions "should be interpreted accordingly." Nevertheless, this claim has been extensively used in Riddell marketing of high school and youth helmets.

Here is just one example taken from the website of Riddell's parent company, Easton Bell, that does not disclose Riddell's role in funding and writing the 2006 study:

"An extensive long-term study by the University of Pittsburgh Medical Center was published in the February 2006 issue of Neurosurgery. The results were impressive: Players wearing the Riddell Revolution football helmet were 31 percent less likely to suffer a concussion than athletes who wore traditional or standard football helmets. For athletes who had never suffered a previous concussion, wearing the Riddell Revolution decreased their relative risk of concussion by 41 percent" Neurosurgery, February 2006, Vol. 58, No. 2. (See http://www.eastonbellsports.com/brands/riddell, accessed Oct. 19, 2011).

The same Easton Bell webpage includes an image of a Riddell Revolution Speed helmet with the claim that "[r]esearch shows a 31 percent reduction in the risk of concussion in players wearing Riddell Revolution helmets when compared to traditionally designed helmets." NEUROSURGERY, FEBRUARY 2006, VOL. 58, NO. 2.

Riddell also uses its reduced risk of concussion claim to sell youth helmets that were not actually tested in the 2006 study of high school football players. For example, Riddell's online store advertises the Riddell Revolution Youth football helmet with the claim that research shows a 31 percent reduction in the risk of concussion when wearing the Riddell Revolution helmet compared to traditional helmets. This webpage does not disclose that the youth helmet was not actually included in the published study:

> "Based on the same technology that made the varsity Riddell Revolution helmet possible—we offer in a Youth version—the Riddell Revolution Youth . . . After an extensive long-term study by the University of Pittsburgh Medical Center was published in the February 2006 issue of Neurosurgery. The results were impressive: research shows a 31 percent reduction in the risk of concussion in players wearing a Riddell Revolution football helmet when compared to traditional helmets." NEUROSURGERY, FEBRUARY 2006, VOL. 58, NO. 2.

Since concussion risk may differ depending on the age group and skill level of players, the results of a single study of high school football players may not be valid for younger children, especially if they wear a different helmet not used in the study. That the youth helmet was not actually tested in the 2006 Neurosurgery study may be a significant omission in such marketing claims used by Riddell and other retailers to sell Revolution youth helmets.

As the official helmet of the National Football League (NFL), Riddell also highlights the use of its products "by the pros" when marketing helmets for high school and younger players. I am concerned by some of the product testimonial claims from one NFL head athletic trainer, Tim Bream of the Chicago Bears, who states in a Riddell Revolution Video News release titled "Riddell Revolution UPMC Media Campaign Highlights":

> "We've had some players who have had ongoing problems with head injury, and we made the switch to the new protective headwear when it came out, at its inception. And these players have had no problems since then, or no repeated concussions."

Bream does not name the players who "had ongoing problems with head injury" before switching to Riddell Revolution helmets. However, the NFL Injury Report website and news articles discussing head injuries suffered by Chicago Bears players during the 2010 football season seem to contradict the claim that wearing the Riddell Revolution helmet prevents all repeated concussions. Three Chicago Bears players who are listed as having head injuries during the 2010 season seem to be wearing Riddell Revolution helmets in press photos. Even if this Riddell Revolution testimonial claim of "no repeated concussions" were true at the time the video was made, one can question whether those who buy the Riddell Revolution helmet for youth or high school players would see similar results of "no repeated concussions."

Riddell uses additional endorsements from this athletic trainer in a January 9, 2006 press release titled Research Shows Riddell Revolution Football Helmet Provides Better Protection Against Concussions (available at: http://www.riddell.com/wp-content/uploads/2006_UPMC_Press_Release_web3.pdf, accessed Oct. 19, 2011) and a 2006 Riddell brochure titled Revolution Helmet Research Findings (available at: http://www.lohud.com/assets/pdf/BH1661391028.PDF, accessed Oct. 19, 2011). In the brochure, Bream states that the "new data [from the 2006 Neurosurgery study] helps our players make an informed choice when deciding which helmet is best for them."

Coaches and athletic equipment managers for youth and high school teams with players who have suffered concussions might also be particularly susceptible to such injury prevention claims. The Orlando Sentinel newspaper's Varsity Sports blog reported on October 17 that one high school football coach and athletic trainer issued a fundraising appeal to buy 60 new Riddell helmets that are "the most-up-to-date . . . concerning concussion reduction technology" since he is concerned about team athletes with multiple concussions. He told the Varsity Sports blog that:

> "In the last three years, we have had eight concussions on the football team . . . What brought us to this point is we have a player who has had a second concussion and of course there is [former South Sumter linebacker] Your highness Morgan [a junior] at Florida Atlantic University but he can't playbecause he has had three concussions in the last two years. We're afraid we are putting our kids at risk. There are recent studies that have shown multiple concussions can lead to a lifetime of medical problems. It's twice the price of the helmets we are wearing now and it's a lot of money to ask a small community to raise but truly, I'm not sure how you cannot afford to get these helmets." (Available at http://blogs.orlandosentinel.com/sports_highschool_varsity/2011/10/17/south-sumter-raising-money-for-new-helmets/, accessed Oct. 19, 2011.)

New Riddell helmets may be very good products. It may also be advisable for this team to replace its old helmets with new headgear. Yet there are still real dangers to overstating the ability of children's sports equipment to prevent brain injury, particularly to coaches and parents of young athletes who have already suffered multiple concussions.

Unfortunately, misleading "anti-concussion" claims appear in advertisements for more than just football helmets. There are other troubling examples of children's sports equipment sold with concussion prevention claims. Although there

is evidence that wearing properly fitted mouth guards reduces the risk of dental injuries, Dr. William Meehan, director of the Sports Concussion Clinic at Children's
Hospital Boston, writes in his 2011 book Kids, Sports, and Concussion: A Guide
for Coaches and Parents that any "effects of [custom mandibular orthotics] and
other mouth guards on concussions remains unknown."

Such uncertainty about the ability of mouth guards to prevent concussions
does not keep some companies from using concussion reduction claims to market mouth guards for youth and high school athletes. The product packaging
for the Brain Pad Lo Pro+ junior mouth guard, which is sold for athletes aged
eleven years and under, prominently states that it "Reduces the Risk of CONCUS-
SIONS!" and "Creates this: BRAIN SAFETY SPACE!" On its Brain Pad Blog,
the company highlights in a banner image the claim "BioMechanically Tested and
Proven to Reduce Concussions Risk by 40 percent!" (see: http://blog.brainpads
.com/, accessed Oct. 19, 2011).

In Brain Pad's online video advertisement titled Head Trainer announces "Zero
concussions with Brain Pad mouth guards!", a head athletic trainer "at one of the
top 5 private [high] schools in the country" who is "responsible for the well-being
of 800 student athletes at the school" states that:

> "We've been using the Brain Pad since 1995. In all those years, whenever
> I go out on the field, especially if somebody has a potential of a concus-
> sion, I always check to see what type of mouth guard they're wearing. And
> I have never, ever seen anybody wearing the Brain Pad and having a con-
> cussion . . . Since 1995, my experience with this mouth guard preventing
> concussions has been absolutely awesome." (see http://www.youtube.com/
> user/brainpads#p/u/3/mtg1EF6LdVQ, accessed Oct. 17, 2011.)

Similar to the Riddell Revolution helmet video described above, this testimonial claim of no concussions among student athletes wearing the Brain Pad mouth
guard seems to imply that those who purchase the product will have similar results. This could lead to young athletes putting themselves at greater risk of head
injury if they believe that they will never suffer a concussion while wearing the
Brain Pad mouth guard.

Another company makes the "Tap Out Youth Mouthguard" for ages 5 to
11 years. The back of the product packaging states that the mouth guard has a
"Concussion Defense System backed by a $30,000 Dental Warranty." Although
this Tap Out mouth guard claim is not as prominent as the previously cited claims
for the Brain Pad mouth guard, it is not clear how the product's "Concussion Defense System" actually protects children from sports-related head injury.

There are also sporting goods companies that sell protective headbands for soccer players with potentially misleading concussion prevention claims. Dr. Meehan notes in Kids, Sports, and Concussion: A Guide for Coaches and Parents that
although many headbands advertise the ability to reduce the risk of concussion,
there is little medical evidence to support this assertion.

The website for ForceField FF headband describes concussions as a problem in soccer and notes that their headband "can come between you and a head injury". The company website states that:

"Research on concussions in soccer has shown that soccer players have concussion rates similar to football and ice hockey . . . The ForceField FF Headband will reduce the risk of head injury when exposed to any type of external force." (See http://www.forcefieldheadbands.com/sportrelated. html accessed Oct. 17, 2011)

Another webpage indicates that the result of wearing the ForceField headband is a "[s]ignificant reduction of the risk of head injuries when exposed to all types of impacts" (available at: http://www.forcefieldheadbands.com/rationale.html, accessed Oct. 17, 2011). The company also markets this headband specifically for use by young children (see: http://www.forcefieldheadbands.com/children.html, accessed Oct. 17, 2011).

Full90 Sports sells other "performance headguards" to protect against concussion in soccer. The company's online store claims the F90 Performance Headguard's "ForceBloc foam reduces impact force by up to 50 percent, meaning fewer concussions overall and a reduction of severity of injury." The company further states that an unnamed "recent study" found that "college players not wearing a Full90 Performance Headguard were 2.65 times more likely to receive a concussion than players that did." (See http://www.full90.com/products/protect/club/ accessed Oct. 19, 2011).

Full 90 Sports' website also includes a product testimonial from a pro soccer player supported by a photo apparently taken moments after he collided with another player. Wearing Full90 headgear, the player looks at his opponent who, not wearing any headgear, appears injured on the ground. The quote accompanying the image is as follows:

"We don't know exactly how much [the headgear] reduced the force of [the impact] but I just thank God . . . I was wearing that thing because I might not be here talking to you had I not worn it. (available at http://www.full90 .com/players/pro/ accessed Oct. 19, 2011. See also image enclosed at end of statement.)

Although this photo and testimonial statement may accurately convey the player's honest belief in the protective properties of Full90 headgear, it is questionable whether there is a reasonable basis to claim that such soccer headgear actually reduces the likelihood and severity of brain injury to any degree.

Such concussion prevention claims used in advertising for a variety of children's sports equipment are very concerning. Paying for a product that does not work as effectively as advertised is bad enough. It is far worse when a product sold for children's use might actually increase the risk of brain injury due to a false sense of security. Enacting the Children's Sports Athletic Equipment Safety Act would discourage companies from misleading coaches, parents, and young athletes.

Unfortunately, one even finds similar, potentially misleading concussion claims in marketing for dietary supplements for children's use. Newport Nutritionals sells Sports Brain Guard, a "[d]aily tri-delivery bioactive protection program" that "help[s] protect your brain from concussion injury" (see http://www.sportsbrainguard.com/ accessed Oct. 19, 2011; See also image at end of statement). Elsewhere on the website, Sports Brain Guard claims to "maximize the brain's ability to heal and reduce inflammation." While this claim may be true, it is not clear that there is enough scientific evidence to date to substantiate that this dietary supplement actually protects the brain from concussion.

Moreover, the net impression of the product's advertising may improperly convey the message that athletes who are concussed or recovering from the lingering effects of concussion can safely "stay in the game" by taking Sports Brain Guard supplements. This "stay in the game" advertising slogan, which is used throughout the product's website, contrasts with the concussion safety and awareness efforts promoted by the CDC and various sports leagues. In fact, the CDC recommends that concussed athletes never return to sports activities "the day of the injury and until a health care professional, experienced in evaluating for concussion, says they are symptom-free and it's OK to return to play" (see http://www.cdc.gov/concussion/what_to_do.html, accessed Oct. 19, 2011).

Yet, despite all this, elsewhere on the site, Newport Nutritionals also prominently announced on the product's homepage that Sports Brain Guard is "Recommended by Dr. Joseph Maroon—Expert in head Injury treatment, Heindl Scholar in Neuroscience, [and] Team Neurosurgeon for the Pittsburg Steelers" (See Sports Brain Guard website from Feb 10, 2011. Internet Archive Wayback Machine. Available at http://web.archive.org/web/20110210114509/http://sportsbrainguard.com/, accessed Oct. 19, 2011). In a separate webpage highlighting his expert endorsement, Maroon states:

> "Over the past 30 years, as a practicing neurosurgeon, I have treated thousands of athletes with sports related concussions—players from the NFL, NHL, NBA, NCAA and all the way down to kids playing youth sports . . . I have personally recommended [this] product, Sports Brain Guard, to athletes at all levels following concussions." (See http://www.sportsbrainguard.com/maroonmsg.aspx, accessed Oct. 19, 2011 and see also image at end of statement)

This kind of testimonial in support of the product from a doctor who has worked in the field of sports concussion is very concerning. It seems to be intended to provide a level of consumer confidence in the efficacy of Sports Brain Guard supplements that does not appear to be justified by scientific data.

Also of great concern, the product website homepage includes a "Notice to Parents" about children and concussion risk that seems to indicate that this product is sold for use by young athletes (See http://www.sportsbrainguard.com/, accessed Oct. 19, 2011; see also image at end of statement). Given the intent seems to be to sell for use by young athletes, it is even more important that the product advertising claims are accurate and supported by scientific evidence.

There are undoubtedly more examples of "anti-concussion" and "concussion reducing" products marketed for children's use. The examples cited above, however, demonstrate that this is already a problem that could become even worse as awareness of sports concussion increases. As we continue to look for the best ways to tackle the problem of sports concussion, we should work to take false advertising out of the game. I hope that responsible sporting goods manufacturers and sports leagues—which are already working to improve concussion awareness among athletes, coaches and parents—will also join in this important effort.

In conclusion, I want to emphasize the very positive role of sports for individuals and our society. Although we now know more about the dangers of concussion, we must not forget how important physical activity and sports are for children. The CDC estimates that only 18 percent of American high school students participate in at least one hour of physical activity a day. That is the amount recommended by the Department of Health and Human Services. Among high school students in New Mexico, only 23 percent are getting the recommended amount of physical activity. This could lead to negative health consequences that last a lifetime.

We know that physically-active youth have lower rates of body fat, better cardio-respiratory fitness, stronger muscles and bones. They also have less anxiety, stress, and depression. As highlighted in HSS's Physical Activities Guidelines for Americans, the bottom line is that the health benefits of physical activity far outweigh the risks of adverse events for almost everyone.

So we need to encourage kids to play sports, to exercise, and to be more physically active. As we learn more about the dangers of concussions for young athletes, we can take steps to make sure sports are played more safely.

STATEMENT OF JEFFREY S. KUTCHER, MD, ASSOCIATE PROFESSOR, UNIVERSITY OF MICHIGAN, DEPARTMENT OF NEUROLOGY; DIRECTOR, MICHIGAN NEUROSPORT; CHAIR, SPORTS NEUROLOGY SECTION, AMERICAN ACADEMY OF NEUROLOGY

. . . Helmets have an extremely important role to play in head injury prevention. Without them, the potential for serious injury would make many of our sports and recreational activities unacceptably risky. In this way, helmets are extremely effective pieces of equipment.

With the introduction of hard-shell helmets, for example, skull fractures from playing football have essentially been eliminated. What helmets do not do well is significantly slow down the contents of the skull when the head is struck or moved suddenly.

Since concussions occur not as a result of the forces experienced by the skull, but by those experienced by the brain, it is extremely unlikely that any helmet can be designed that will prevent concussions to the same significant degree that they have been shown to prevent skull fractures.

Currently, there are no convincing data in the published medical literature that show any particular helmet being better than any other at preventing sports concussion. Such data is hard to collect, grant you, for two main reasons.

First, given the many variables that exist in the athletic population and the varied exposure to impacts, it is extremely difficult to perform a randomized, controlled clinical trial on similar populations of athletes. Second, given that concussion is a clinical diagnosis with no available reference standard or diagnostic test, any study of concussion is significantly limited by the ambiguity of the very clinical outcome that is being studied.

For these same reasons, there are no published data supporting the idea that other types of protective equipment, such as mouth guards or soccer headbands, prevent concussion. Moreover, in sports such as soccer, where protective headgear is the exception rather than the rule, I have seen the use of headgear result in athletes altering their playing style in the wrong direction as their newfound sense of protection encourages more physically aggressive play.

Every week, I am asked in my clinic by patients, parents, and coaches about the claims they hear and what equipment they should buy to prevent concussions. The simple truth is that no current helmet, mouth guard, headband, or other piece of equipment can significantly prevent concussions from occurring. They occur as the result of the nature of our sports.

Concussion prevention is much more about teaching proper technique, playing by the rules, and limiting the overall dose of impacts. The potential harm that I see caused by products that claim to prevent concussion when they do not is far more than simply the financial harm of paying more for something that isn't likely to work as claimed. It is the harm that comes from having a false sense of security, from not understanding how the injury occurs, and what can actually be done to prevent it.

The public deserves to know that equipment has a significant, but inherently limited ability to prevent concussion. There is still a tremendous amount yet to be learned about the nature of concussions and their possible effects on brain health. In the interim, I am deeply encouraged by today's hearing and honored to be included in the efforts of the Committee as we work together for the safety of our athletes . . .

Equipment Limitations

Helmets have an extremely important role to play in head injury prevention. Without them, the potential for bone fracture or intracranial injury would make many of our sports and recreational activities unacceptably risky. In this way, helmets are extremely effective pieces of equipment. With the introduction of hard-shell helmets, for example, skull fractures and resulting deaths from playing football have essentially been eliminated. What helmets do not do well is significantly slow down the contents of the skull when the head is struck or moves suddenly. Since concussions occur not as a result of the forces experienced by the skull, but by those experienced by the brain, it is extremely unlikely that any helmet can be designed that will prevent concussions to the same significant degree that they have been shown to prevent skull fractures.

Currently, there is no data in the published medical literature that shows any particular helmet being better than any other at preventing sports concussions. Such data is hard to collect for two main reasons: First, given the many variables that exist in the athletic population and the varied exposure to impacts, it is extremely difficult to perform a randomized, controlled, clinical trial on similar populations of athletes. Second, given that concussion is a clinical diagnosis, with no available reference standard or diagnostic test, any study of concussion is significantly limited by the ambiguity of the very clinical outcome that is being studied.

For these same reasons, there are no published data supporting the idea that other types of protective equipment, such as mouth guards or soccer headbands, prevent concussion. Moreover, in sports such as soccer, where protective headgear is the exception rather than the rule, I have seen the use of headgear result in athletes altering their playing style in the wrong direction, as their newfound sense of protection encourages more physically aggressive play.

While clinical data that speaks to concussion prevention is hard to generate, there are many extremely well performed laboratory studies that provide excellent data on the amount of force a helmet allows to get through to a model brain in a mechanical head. This does not mean that these data can be used to construct an estimate of concussion risk. Concussions do not occur at a particular force threshold. They occur across a wide range of forces and are dependent on the complex and variable physiological nature of each individual's brain.

The Potential Harm of Misinformation

With the increased public awareness of an injury that occurs frequently in children and may produce significant negative long-term health outcomes, it is not surprising that the marketplace for products designed to prevent concussions is a busy one. Every week I am asked by patients, parents, and coaches about the claims they hear and what equipment they should buy to prevent concussions. I wish there was such a product on the market. The simple truth is that no current helmet, mouth guard, headband, or other piece of equipment can significantly prevent concussions from occurring. They occur as the result of the nature of sports. Concussion prevention is much more about teaching proper technique, playing by the rules, and limiting the overall dose of impacts. Preventing bad outcomes and long-term damage, meanwhile, is clearly about recognizing the injury when it occurs, removing that athlete from participation, and allowing for appropriate recovery before they return.

The potential harm that I see being caused by products that claim to prevent concussion when they do not is far more than simply the financial harm of paying more for something that isn't likely to work as claimed. It is the harm that comes from having a false sense of security, from not understanding how the injury occurs and what can actually be done to prevent it. This issue is a growing public concern, and rightly so. The public deserves to know that equipment has a significant, but inherently limited, ability to prevent concussions. For the health of all athletes, we must see that each player, parent, and coach becomes educated on concussion, including the use of proper technique, the need for reporting the injury, and the importance of allowing for a full recovery before returning.

There is still a tremendous amount yet to be learned about the nature of concussions and their possible effects on brain health. In the interim, I am deeply encouraged by today's hearing and honored to be included in the efforts of the Committee as we work together for the safety of our athletes . . .

PREPARED STATEMENT OF MIKE OLIVER, EXECUTIVE DIRECTOR AND LEGAL COUNSEL, THE NATIONAL OPERATING COMMITTEE ON STANDARDS FOR ATHLETIC EQUIPMENT (NOCSAE)

. . . While helmets certified to NOCSAE standards play an incredibly important role in protecting athletes in the field of play, improved protective equipment is not the only solution to providing better protection against concussion. Prevention, diagnosis, treatment, and management decisions about when athletes should return to play are equally important, and prevention can be enhanced by enforcing the rules of play in a particular sport.

Teaching and enforcing proper tackling techniques, which include not using the head as a weapon or primary contact point. These types of changes can make an immediate and likely measurable impact on the number and severity of concussions.

Teaching athletes and active children at all ages that the signs and symptoms of a potential concussion should not be ignored, and should be followed up with an evaluation by someone properly trained and skilled in evaluating concussions.

Adopting and enforcing return to play criteria that will prevent an athlete from returning to play until a complete and objective evaluation is completed.

Helping parents, coaches, and players understand that although helmets provide a substantial level of protection, no helmet can prevent all head injuries, including concussions . . .

. . . Senator Udall. Thank you, Mr. Chairman.

Dr. Kutcher, your testimony states, and I think you said this also orally here, there is no data in the published medical literature that shows any particular helmet being better than any other at preventing sports concussions.

Last year, however, the CEO of Riddell testified before a different Congressional committee that Riddell has "independent, peer-reviewed, published research in the medical journal Neurosurgery, February 2006, showing that Revolution"—that is the name of their helmet—"reduces the risk of concussions by 31 percent when compared to traditional helmets."

One of the authors of the 2006 study told the New York Times earlier this year that he disagreed with Riddell's marketing the 31 percent figure without acknowledging its limitations. Yet Riddell has extensively used this concussion safety claim in its marketing, and here is just one example with this poster that is behind me.

[An image of the poster follows:]

This is an example taken today from the website of Riddell's parent company, and I think you can read that.

The Chairman. I can't read it.

Senator Udall. Do you think this single 2006 study provides a reasonable basis for Riddell to claim that the research shows that Revolution helmets reduce the risk of concussion by 31 percent compared to the traditional helmets?

Dr. Kutcher. No, I do not. I am aware of this study, and what I said was that there is no significant data to make that claim in the literature. I know there is data. That study is in the literature.

There are mainly two problems with that study. First is the quality of the study itself, how it was set up in trying to look at two different populations, one wearing a certain helmet, one wearing another kind of helmet. You want those populations to be as equal as possible, other than which helmet they are wearing. And that was not very well done in that study, to the point where I would not really consider the study design to be acceptable scientific protocol.

The second main critique is that the 31 percent figure is a relative percent change. So the two populations, the one that had the old helmet had a 7.6 percent concussion rate over the study period. The new helmet had a 5.3 percent rate. The change was 2.6 percent. The absolute percent change. That is a relative percent change.

But when you put the 31 percent figure in front of people like that, they are going to think that there are 31 percent less concussions. Well, actually, it is 2.6 percent and that amount, given the study limitations, would more than account for sort of that noise in the data.

Senator Udall. And you can see why a parent who would be concerned about concussions with all the awareness, increasing awareness that is out there would see something like this and see 31 percent and think, "I am going to get a really protective helmet for my child." And really, what we are talking about is something that is very, very misleading.

Dr. Kutcher. Well, I can see that, and I do see that every week in my clinic. I see patients coming in with their parents saying they want to buy the new helmet. This is the concussion helmet. What do you think about it? That is a very real conversation I have all the time.

Senator Udall. And they are asking you that question over and over again?

Dr. Kutcher. Correct.

Senator Udall. And typically, what do you tell them? And then, do you know what they do afterwards?

Dr. Kutcher. So my advice is the most important thing is to have a new helmet if you can get one. In other words, try to avoid the reconditioning situation where you don't know whether the helmet is still up to standards provided by NOCSAE.

But fit is really important. Make sure the helmet is fit correctly. And then, after that, I say look at the different manufacturers, and if money is not an option, buy the highest one on the line because what is lost in this conversation is you can't have a concussion without force, right? But force is not the only thing going on here, right?

So if I took 100 athletes or 100 people and gave them the same blow to the head I am going to get 100 different responses. So to say that concussion is the issue is ignoring the fact that it is forces acting on a brain that is very individualized and very dynamic.

So, at the end of the day, if I am going to pick between a helmet that gets the least amount of force through versus one that gets a little more force through, I am going to pick the one that gets the least amount of force through. I think that is a fair thing to say. But to say that it is going to prevent concussion is not understanding the whole complexity of the issue.

Senator Udall. Thank you very much . . .

. . . Dr. McKee. Well, I believe there is no clear evidence that any mouth guard or chin guard reduces either the rate or the severity of concussions. So I would have great objection to this claim.

The only thing that I am aware that mouth guards and chin guards do is they reduce oral and facial, dental, dental injuries. But the nature of concussion would not be improved by the use of a mouth guard.

Senator Udall. I know you weren't able to see the one I was holding up, and I think it has been produced down there just in case you see anything else on it you wanted to comment on.

Dr. Kutcher. I agree on that.

Senator Udall. Yes, please?

Dr. Kutcher. I don't know what "brain safety space" really means. That term— that is little alarming, really.

Senator Udall. Well, there is a diagram on it.

Dr. Kutcher. Yes, I see it.

Senator Udall. You can see it. There is a diagram, and it shows a space, and it says "creates brain"—I believe specifically it says, "creates"—what is the term it uses? "Creates brain safety space."

Dr. Kutcher. Again, the idea from some of the work that has been done with accelerometers and helmets of football players and seeing at what forces they end up having clinically diagnosed concussions, those concussions are occurring over a wide range of forces.

There are 15-g hits that do it. There are 115-g hits that don't, right? And so, if you are taking amount of force that is 115 and you are reducing it to 110 or so—I don't want to get the numbers wrong—because of a mouth guard, you might be reducing the forces a little bit if the hit is coming from this way, but concussions are occurring on a spectrum of forces that that won't address.

Senator Udall. I know Ms. Ball mentioned headbands in soccer, and I want to ask, Dr. Kutcher, you about this one. You discuss in your testimony the potential harm from creating a false sense of security when companies falsely claim that products prevent concussions.

This is not just about helmets, and it is not just about football. Here is another example. This is a protective headband sold to soccer players and other athletes. Here is an image taken from this company's website that says, "This can come between you and a head injury."

Does this type of advertising for a protective headband trouble you? Is there a danger that a young athlete might put himself or herself at greater risk of injury if they believe that this headband will come between them and a head injury?

Dr. Kutcher. I do believe there is a problem there. This type of advertising is a little more vague because it just mentions head injury and not concussion. So you could make an argument that perhaps there is a mechanism there to prevent some superficial lacerations and bruising and that kind of a thing. But for concussion, I don't believe that—well, there is no data that supports that they decrease the risk of concussion.

I have seen in my own practice, as I testified, athletes who have become more aggressive and have actually injured themselves and others because they have the headband on. They go up and they head the ball more. They get involved in head-to-head hits more when they would not have done that without the equipment before . . .

Source: "Concussions and the Marketing of Sports Equipment." Hearing before the Committee on Commerce, Science, and Transportation. United States Senate, 112th Congress, 1st Session, October 19, 2011. S. Hrg. 112–324. Washington, DC: Government Printing Office, 2012.

Opinion of the United States Court of Appeals for the Third Circuit Regarding National Football League Players Concussion Litigation

Concussion is a relatively common injury in American football. Evidence suggests that concussions have a cumulative effect—the more you sustain, the greater your risk of developing long-term health and cognitive problems. Many former players from the National Football League are upset because they were not informed of the potential cumulative effects during their playing years, and thus were unable to factor this into their decisions about if and when to return to football after sustaining concussions. In a federal lawsuit, they contended that the NFL, its medical committee, and its medical director purposely argued that concussion had no cumulative effect, showing their own results that were in contrast with the bulk of evidence being reported elsewhere. Below are some excerpts from the opinion of one of the appeals.

IN RE: NATIONAL FOOTBALL LEAGUE PLAYERS CONCUSSION INJURY LITIGATION

Opinion of the Court

Introduction

The National Football League ("NFL") has agreed to resolve lawsuits brought by former players who alleged that the NFL failed to inform them of and protect them from the risks of concussions in football. The District Court approved a class action settlement that covered over 20,000 retired players and released all concussion-related claims against the NFL. Objectors have appealed that decision, arguing that class certification was improper and that the settlement was unfair. But after thorough review, we conclude that the District Court was right to certify the class and approve the settlement. Thus we affirm its decision in full.

II. Background

A. CONCUSSION SUITS ARE BROUGHT AGAINST THE NFL

In July 2011, 73 former professional football players sued the NFL and Riddell, Inc. in the Superior Court of California. Compl., *Maxwell v. Nat'l Football League*, No. BC465842 (Cal. Super. Ct. July 19, 2011). The retired players alleged that the NFL failed to take reasonable actions to protect them from the chronic risks of head injuries in football. The players also claimed that Riddell, a manufacturer of sports equipment, should be liable for the defective design of helmets.

The NFL removed the case to federal court on the ground that the players' claims under state law were preempted by federal labor law. More lawsuits by retired players followed and the NFL moved under 28 U.S.C. § 1407 to consolidate the pending suits before a single judge for pretrial proceedings. In January 2012, the Judicial Panel on Multidistrict Litigation consolidated these cases before Judge Anita B. Brody in the Eastern District of Pennsylvania as a multidistrict litigation ("MDL"). *In re: Nat'l Football League Players' Concussion Injury Litig.*, 842 F. Supp. 2d 1378 (J.P.M.L. 2012). Since consolidation, 5,000 players have filed over 300 similar lawsuits against the NFL and Riddell.1 Our appeal only concerns the claims against the NFL.

There is also a pending class action against the National Collegiate Athletic Association ("NCAA") over its handling of head injuries. In January 2016, the District Court overseeing the action preliminarily certified the class and approved a settlement subject to certain revisions. *In re: Nat'l Collegiate Athletic Ass'n Student-Athlete Concussion Injury Litig.*, No. 13–9116, 2016 WL 305380 (N.D. Ill. Jan. 26, 2016). Under the settlement, the NCAA will pay $70 million to create a medical monitoring fund to screen current and former collegiate athletes for brain trauma.

To manage the litigation, the District Court appointed co-lead class counsel, a Steering Committee, and an Executive Committee. The Steering Committee was charged with performing or delegating all necessary pretrial tasks and the smaller Executive Committee was responsible for the overall coordination of the proceedings. The Court also ordered plaintiffs to submit a Master Administrative Long-Form Complaint and a Master Administrative Class Action Complaint to supersede the numerous then-pending complaints.

The Master Complaints tracked many of the allegations from the first lawsuits. Football puts players at risk of repetitive brain trauma and injury because they suffer concussive and sub-concussive hits during the game and at practice (sub-concussive hits fall below the threshold for a concussion but are still associated with brain damage). Plaintiffs alleged that the NFL had a duty to provide players with rules and information to protect them from the health risks—both short and long-term—of brain injury, including Alzheimer's disease, dementia, depression, deficits in cognitive functioning, reduced processing speed, loss of memory, sleeplessness, mood swings, personality changes, and a recently identified degenerative disease called chronic traumatic encephalopathy (commonly referred to as "CTE").

Because CTE figures prominently in this appeal, some background on this condition is in order. It was first identified in 2002 based on analysis of the brain tissue of deceased NFL players, including Mike Webster, Terry Long, Andre Waters, and Justin Strzelczyk. CTE involves the build-up of "tau protein" in the brain, a result associated with repetitive head trauma. Medical personnel have examined approximately 200 brains with CTE as of 2015, in large part because it is only diagnosable post-mortem. That diagnosis requires examining sections of a person's brain under a microscope to see if abnormal tau proteins are present and, if so, whether they occur in the unique pattern associated with CTE. Plaintiffs alleged that CTE affects mood and behavior, causing headaches, aggression, depression, and an increased risk of suicide. They also stated that memory loss, dementia, loss of attention and concentration, and impairment of language are associated with CTE.

The theme of the allegations was that, despite the NFL's awareness of the risks of repetitive head trauma, the League ignored, minimized, or outright suppressed information concerning the link between that trauma and cognitive damage. For example, in 1994 the NFL created the Mild Traumatic Brain Injury Committee to study the effects of head injuries. Per the plaintiffs, the Committee was at the forefront of a disinformation campaign that disseminated "junk science" denying the link between head injuries and cognitive disorders. Based on the allegations against the NFL, plaintiffs asserted claims for negligence, medical monitoring, fraudulent concealment, fraud, negligent misrepresentation, negligent hiring, negligent retention, wrongful death and survival, civil conspiracy, and loss of consortium.

After plaintiffs filed the Master Complaints, the NFL moved to dismiss, arguing that federal labor law preempted the state law claims. Indeed, § 301 of the Labor Management Relations Act preempts state law claims that are "substantially dependent" on the terms of a labor agreement. *Int'l Bhd. of Elec. Workers v. Hechler*, 481 U.S. 851, 852–53 (1987). The NFL claimed that resolution of plaintiffs' claims depended upon the interpretation of Collective Bargaining Agreements ("CBAs") in place between the retired players and the NFL.2 If the CBAs do preempt plaintiffs' claims, they must arbitrate those claims per mandatory arbitration provisions in the CBAs. Plaintiffs responded that their negligence and fraud claims would not require federal courts to interpret the CBAs and in any event the CBAs did not cover all retired players.2

After the NFL removed some of the early concussion-related lawsuits from state courts, several district courts accepted this preemption argument as a basis for denying requests to remand the cases. See, e.g., *Smith v. Nat'l Football League Players Ass'n*, No. 14–1559, 2014 WL 6776306, at *9 (E.D. Mo. Dec. 2, 2014); *Duerson v. Nat'l Football League, Inc.*, No. 12–2513, 2012 WL 1658353, at *6 (N.D. Ill. May 11, 2012); *but see Green v. Arizona Cardinals Football Club LLC*, 21 F. Supp. 3d 1020, 1030 (E.D. Mo. 2014) (finding that concussion-related claims did not depend on interpretation of CBAs and granting motion to remand).

B. THE PARTIES REACH A SETTLEMENT

On July 8, 2013, while the NFL's motion to dismiss was pending, the District Court ordered the parties to mediate and appointed a mediator. On August 29, 2013, after two months of negotiations and more than twelve full days of formal mediation, the parties agreed to a settlement in principle and signed a term sheet. It provided $765 million to fund medical exams and offer compensation for player injuries. The proposed settlement would resolve the claims of all retired players against the NFL related to head injuries.

In January 2014, after more negotiations, class counsel filed in the District Court a class action complaint and sought preliminary class certification and preliminary approval of the settlement. The Court denied the motion because it had doubts that the capped fund for paying claims would be sufficient. *In re Nat'l Football League Players' Concussion Injury Litig.*, 961 F. Supp. 2d 708, 715 (E.D. Pa. 2014). It appointed a Special Master to assist with making financial forecasts and, five months later, the parties reached a revised settlement that uncapped the fund for compensating retired players.

Class counsel filed a second motion for preliminary class certification and preliminary approval in June 2014. The District Court granted the motion, preliminarily approved the settlement, conditionally certified the class, approved classwide notice, and scheduled a final fairness hearing. *In re Nat'l Football League Players' Concussion Injury Litig.*, 301 F.R.D. 191 (E.D. Pa. 2014). Seven players petitioned for interlocutory review. *See* Fed. R. Civ. P. 23(f) ("A court of appeals may permit an appeal from an order granting or denying class-action certification under this rule if a petition for permission to appeal is filed with the circuit clerk within 14 days after the order is entered."). In September 2014, we denied the petition, later explaining over a dissent that we lacked jurisdiction because the District Court's order preliminarily certifying the class was not an "order granting or denying class-action certification." *In re Nat'l Football League Players' Concussion Injury Litig.*, 775 F.3d 570, 571–72 (3d Cir. 2014).

Following preliminary certification, potential class members had 90 days to object or opt out of the settlement. Class counsel then moved for final class certification and settlement approval. On November 19, 2014, the District Court held a day-long fairness hearing and heard argument from class counsel, the NFL, and several objectors who voiced concerns against the settlement. After the hearing, the Court proposed several changes to benefit class members. The parties agreed to the proposed changes and submitted an amended settlement in February 2015.

On April 22, 2015, the Court granted the motion for class certification and final approval of the amended settlement, that grant explained in a 123-page opinion. *In re Nat'l Football League Players' Concussion Injury Litig.*, 307 F.R.D. 351 (E.D. Pa. 2015). Objectors filed 12 separate appeals that were consolidated into this single appeal before us now.

C. THE PROPOSED SETTLEMENT

The settlement has three components: (1) an uncapped Monetary Award Fund that provides compensation for retired players who submit proof of certain diagnoses; (2) a $75 million Baseline Assessment Program that provides eligible retired players with free baseline assessment examinations of their objective neurological functioning; and (3) a $10 million Education Fund to instruct football players about injury prevention.

1. MONETARY AWARD FUND

Under the settlement, retired players or their beneficiaries are compensated for developing one of several neurocognitive and neuromuscular impairments or "Qualifying Diagnoses." By "retired players," we mean players who retired from playing NFL football before the preliminary approval of the class settlement on July 7, 2014. The settlement recognizes six Qualifying Diagnoses: (1) Level 1.5 Neurocognitive Impairment; (2) Level 2 Neurocognitive Impairment;3 (3) Alzheimer's Disease; (4) Parkinson's Disease; (5) Amyotrophic Lateral Sclerosis ("ALS"); and (6) Death with CTE provided the player died before final approval of the settlement on April 22, 2015. A retired player does not need to show that his time in the NFL caused the onset of the Qualifying Diagnosis.3 Levels 1.5 and 2 Neurocognitive Impairment require a decline in cognitive function and a loss of functional capabilities, such as the ability to hold a job, and correspond with clinical definitions of mild and moderate dementia.

A Qualifying Diagnosis entitles a retired player to a maximum monetary award:

Qualifying diagnosis	Maximum award
Level 1.5 Neurocognitive Impairment	$1.5 Million
Level 2 Neurocognitive Impairment	$3 Million
Parkinson's Disease	$3.5 Million
Alzheimer's Disease	$3.5 Million
Death with CTE	$4 Million
ALS	$5 Million

This award is subject to several offsets, that is, awards decrease: (1) as the age at which a retired player is diagnosed increases; (2) if the retired player played fewer than five eligible seasons; (3) if the player did not have a baseline assessment examination; and (4) if the player suffered a severe traumatic brain injury or stroke unrelated to NFL play.

To collect from the Fund, a class member must register with the claims administrator within 180 days of receiving notice that the settlement has been approved. This deadline can be excused for good cause. The class member then must submit a claims package to the administrator no later than two years after the date of the Qualifying Diagnosis or within two years after the supplemental notice is posted on the settlement website, whichever is later. This deadline can be excused for substantial hardship. The claims package must include a certification by the diagnosing physician and supporting medical records. The claims administrator will notify the class member within 60 days if he is entitled to an award. The class member, class counsel, and the NFL have the right to appeal an award determination. To do so, a class member must submit a $1,000 fee, which is refunded if the appeal is successful and can be waived for financial hardship. A fee is not required for the NFL and class counsel to appeal, though the NFL must act in good faith when appealing award determinations.

The Monetary Award Fund is uncapped and will remain in place for 65 years. Every retired player who timely registers and qualifies during the lifespan of the settlement will receive an award. If, after receiving an initial award, a retired player receives a more serious Qualifying Diagnosis, he may receive a supplemental award.

2. BASELINE ASSESSMENT PROGRAM

Any retired player who has played at least half of an eligible season can receive a baseline assessment examination. It consists of a neurological examination performed by credentialed and licensed physicians selected by a court-appointed administrator. Qualified providers may diagnose retired players with Level 1, 1.5, or 2 Neurocognitive Impairment. The results of the examinations can also be compared with any future tests to determine whether a retired player's cognitive abilities have deteriorated.

Baseline Assessment Program funds will also provide Baseline Assessment Program Supplemental Benefits. Retired players diagnosed with Level 1 Neurocognitive Impairment—evidencing some objective decline in cognitive function but not yet early dementia—are eligible to receive medical benefits, including further testing, treatment, counseling, and pharmaceutical coverage.

The Baseline Assessment Program lasts for 10 years. All retired players who seek and are eligible for a baseline assessment examination receive one notwithstanding the $75 million cap. Every eligible retired player age 43 or over must take a baseline assessment examination within two years of the Program's start-up. Every eligible retired player younger than age 43 must do so before the end of the program or by his 45th birthday, whichever comes first.

3. EDUCATION FUND

The Education Fund is a $10 million fund to promote safety and injury prevention in football. The purpose is to promote safety-related initiatives in youth football and educate retired players about their medical and disability benefits under the CBA. Class counsel and the NFL, with input from the retired players, will propose specific educational initiatives for the District Court's approval.

4. THE PROPOSED CLASS

All living NFL football players who retired from playing professional football before July 7, 2014, as well as their representative claimants and derivative claimants, comprise the proposed class. Representative claimants are those duly authorized by law to assert the claims of deceased, legally incapacitated, or incompetent retired players. Derivative claimants are those, such as parents, spouses, or dependent children, who have some legal right to the income of retired players. Even though the proposed class consists of more than just retired players, we use the terms "class members" and "retired players" interchangeably.

The proposed class contains two subclasses based on a retired players' injuries as of the preliminary approval date. Subclass 1 consists of retired players who were not diagnosed with a Qualifying Diagnosis prior to July 7, 2014, and their representative and derivative claimants. Put another way, subclass 1 includes retired players who have no currently known injuries that would be compensated under the settlement. Subclass 2 consists of retired players who were diagnosed with a Qualifying Diagnosis prior to July 7, 2014, and their representative claimants and derivative claimants. Translated, subclass 2 includes retired players who are currently injured and will receive an immediate monetary award under the settlement. The NFL estimates that the total population of retired players is 21,070. Of this, 28% are expected to be diagnosed with a compensable disease. The remaining 72% are not expected to develop a compensable disease during their lifetime.

Class members release all claims and actions against the NFL "arising out of, or relating to, head, brain and/or cognitive injury, as well as any injuries arising out of, or relating to, concussions and/or sub-concussive events," including claims relating to CTE. The releases do not compromise the benefits that retired players are entitled to receive under the CBAs, nor do they compromise their retirement benefits, disability benefits, and health insurance.

Of the over 20,000 estimated class members (the NFL states that the number exceeds 21,000), 234 initially asked to opt out from the settlement and 205 class members joined 83 written objections submitted to the District Court. Before the fairness hearing, 26 of the 234 opt-outs sought readmission to the class. After the District Court granted final approval, another 6 opt-outs sought readmission. This leaves 202 current opt-outs, of which class counsel notes only 169 were timely filed.

. . . B. GIRSH & PRUDENTIAL FACTORS

In *Girsh v. Jepson*, we noted nine factors to be considered when determining the fairness of a proposed settlement:

- The complexity, expense and likely duration of the litigation; (2) the reaction of the class to the settlement; (3) the stage of the proceedings and the amount of discovery completed; (4) the risks of establishing liability; (5) the risks of establishing damages; (6) the risks of maintaining the class action through the trial; (7) the ability of the defendants to withstand a greater judgment; (8) the range of reasonableness of the settlement fund in light of the best possible recovery; and (9) the range of reasonableness of the settlement fund to a possible recovery in light of all the attendant risks of litigation.

521 F.2d 153, 157 (3d Cir. 1975) (internal quotation marks and ellipses omitted). "The settling parties bear the burden of proving that the *Girsh* factors weigh in favor of approval of the settlement." *In re Pet Food Prods.*, 629 F.3d at 350. A district court's findings under the *Girsh* test are those of fact. Unless clearly erroneous, they are upheld. *Id.*

Later, in *Prudential Insurance* we held that, because of a "sea-change in the nature of class actions," it might be useful to expand the *Girsh* factors to include several permissive and non-exhaustive factors:

[1] The maturity of the underlying substantive issues, as measured by experience in adjudicating individual actions, the development of scientific knowledge, the extent of discovery on the merits, and other factors that bear on the ability to assess the probable outcome of a trial on the merits of liability and individual damages; [2] the existence and probable outcome of claims by other classes and subclasses; [3] the comparison between the results achieved by the settlement for individual class or subclass members and the results achieved—or likely to be achieved—for other claimants; [4] whether class or subclass members are accorded the right to opt out of the settlement; [5] whether any provisions for attorneys' fees are reasonable; and [6] whether the procedure for processing individual claims under the settlement is fair and reasonable.

148 F.3d at 323. "Unlike the *Girsh* factors, each of which the district court must consider before approving a class settlement, the *Prudential* considerations are just that, prudential." *In re Baby Prods.*, 708 F.3d at 174.

The District Court in our case went through the *Girsh* factors and the relevant *Prudential* factors in great detail before concluding that the terms of the settlement were fair, reasonable, and adequate. *In re Nat'l Football League Players' Concussion Injury Litig.*, 307 F.R.D. at 388–96. Objectors try to challenge the District Court's analysis in several ways, but none convinces us.

1. COMPLEXITY, EXPENSE, AND LIKELY DURATION OF THE LITIGATION

"The first factor 'captures the probable costs, in both time and money, of continued litigation.'" *Warfarin*, 391 F.3d at 535–36 (quoting *Cendant*, 264 F.3d at 233). The District Court concluded that the probable costs of continued litigation in the MDL were significant and that this factor weighed in favor of approving the settlement. *In re Nat'l Football League Players' Concussion Injury Litig.*,

307 F.R.D. at 388–89. Some objectors assert that the District Court overestimated the costs of continued litigation because the negligence and fraud claims were "straightforward." This is not the case. Over 5,000 retired NFL players in the MDL alleged a multi-decade fraud by the NFL, and litigating these claims would have been an enormous undertaking. The discovery needed to prove the NFL's fraudulent concealment of the risks of concussions was extensive. The District Court would then resolve many issues of causation and medical science. Finally, if the cases did not settle or were not dismissed, individual suits would be remanded to district courts throughout the country for trial. We agree with the District Court that the expense of this process weighs strongly in the settlement's favor.

2. REACTION OF THE CLASS TO THE SETTLEMENT

"The second *Girsh* factor 'attempts to gauge whether members of the class support the settlement.'" *Warfarin*, 391 F.3d at 536 (quoting *Prudential*, 148 F.3d at 318). As noted, the case began with a class of approximately 20,000 retired players, of which 5,000 are currently represented by counsel in the MDL proceedings. Notice of the settlement reached an estimated 90% of those players through direct mail and secondary publications (in addition to the extensive national media coverage of this case). As of 10 days before the fairness hearing, more than 5,200 class members had signed up to receive additional information about the settlement and the settlement website had more than 64,000 unique visitors. With all this attention, only approximately 1% of class members objected and approximately 1% of class members opted out. We agree with the District Court that these figures weigh in favor of settlement approval. *In re Nat'l Football League Players' Concussion Injury Litig.*, 307 F.R.D. at 389.

Some note that the percentage of objectors was even lower in *GM Trucks*, a case where we declined to approve a settlement. There, "[o]f approximately 5.7 million class members, 6,450 owners objected and 5,203 opted out." *GM Trucks*, 55 F.3d at 813 n.32. But in *GM* we looked past the low objection rate because there were "other indications that the class reaction to the suit was quite negative," including our concern that the passive victims of a product defect lacked "adequate interest and information to voice objections." *Id.* at 813. Those concerns are not present here. By the time of the settlement, many of the retired players in this class already had counsel and had sued the NFL, suggesting that their claims were valuable enough to pursue in court and that the players were informed enough to evaluate the settlement.12

Others argue that we cannot rely on the reaction of the class because the class notice was "problematic." They claim that the notice may have misled class members about compensation for those with a post-mortem CTE diagnosis. But the District Court explained that the class notice was clear that only some cases of CTE would be compensated. *In re Nat'l Football League Players' Concussion Injury Litig.*, 307 F.R.D. at 383–84.

3. STAGE OF THE PROCEEDINGS AND AMOUNT OF DISCOVERY COMPLETED

"The third *Girsh* factor 'captures the degree of case development that class counsel [had] accomplished prior to settlement. Through this lens, courts can determine whether counsel had an adequate appreciation of the merits of the case before negotiating.'" *Warfarin*, 391 F.3d at 537 (quoting *Cendant*, 264 F.3d at 235).

The District Court concluded that class counsel adequately evaluated the merits of the preemption and causation issues through informal discovery, and, after ten months of settlement negotiations, the stage of the proceedings weighed in favor of settlement approval. *In re Nat'l Football League Players' Concussion Injury Litig.*, 307 F.R.D. at 390. Objectors claim that the lack of formal discovery in this matter should have weighed more heavily against settlement. As with the presumption of fairness, formal discovery is not a requirement for the third *Girsh* factor. What matters is not the amount or type of discovery class counsel pursued, but whether they had developed enough information about the case to appreciate sufficiently the value of the claims. Moreover, requiring parties to conduct formal discovery before reaching a proposed class settlement would take a valuable bargaining chip—the costs of formal discovery itself—off the table during negotiations. This could deter the early settlement of disputes.

4. RISKS OF ESTABLISHING LIABILITY AND DAMAGES

"The fourth and fifth *Girsh* factors survey the possible risks of litigation in order to balance the likelihood of success and the potential damage award if the case were taken to trial against the benefits of an immediate settlement." *Prudential*, 148 F.3d at 319. We concur with the District Court that this factor weighed in favor of settlement because class members "face[d] stiff challenges surmounting the issues of preemption and causation." *In re Nat'l Football League Players' Concussion Injury Litig.*, 307 F.R.D. at 391.

To start, if the NFL were to prevail in its motion to dismiss on the issue of federal labor law preemption, "many, if not all," of the class members' claims would be dismissed. *Id.* Objectors claim the District Court misjudged the risks of establishing liability and damages on this front. They argue that the NFL's preemption defense would not apply to all class members because there were no CBAs in effect before 1968 and between 1987 and 1993. But even if there were a small subset of players unaffected by the preemption defense, the defense still had the capability of denying relief to the majority of class members, and this weighs in favor of approving the settlement.

As for causation, the District Court noted that retired players would need to show both general causation (that repetitive head trauma is capable of causing ALS, Alzheimer's, and the like), and specific causation (that the brain trauma suffered by a particular player, in fact, caused his specific impairments). *In re Nat'l Football League Players' Concussion Injury Litig.*, 307 F.R.D. at 393. With general causation, the Court found that even though "[a] consensus is emerging that repetitive mild brain injury is associated with the Qualifying Diagnoses," the "available research is not nearly robust enough to discount the risks" of litigation. *Id.* And specific causation would be even more troublesome because a player would need to distinguish the effect of hits he took during his NFL career from the effect of those he received in high school football, college football, or other contact sports. Objectors argue that the District Court put too little faith in the ability of the class to show causation because the NFL has admitted that concussions can lead to long-term problems and formal discovery could disclose that it fraudulently concealed the risks of concussions. But neither of these points is particularly helpful for overcoming the general and specific causation hurdles the District Court identified.

5. RISKS OF MAINTAINING CLASS ACTION THROUGH TRIAL

The District Court found that the likelihood of obtaining and keeping a class certification if the action were to proceed to trial weighed in favor of approving the settlement, but it deserved only minimal consideration. *Id.* at 394. This was correct. In a settlement class, this factor becomes essentially "toothless" because " 'a district court need not inquire whether the case, if tried, would present intractable management problems[,] . . . for the proposal is that there be no trial.'" *Prudential*, 148 F.3d at 321 (quoting *Amchem*, 521 U.S. at 620).

6. ABILITY OF DEFENDANTS TO WITHSTAND A GREATER JUDGMENT

The seventh *Girsh* factor is most relevant when the defendant's professed inability to pay is used to justify the amount of the settlement. In the case of the NFL, the District Court found this factor neutral because the NFL did not cite potential financial instability as justification for the settlement's size. *In re Nat'l Football League Players' Concussion Injury Litig.*, 307 F.R.D. at 394. In fact, it agreed to uncap the Monetary Award Fund and is thus duty bound to pay every compensable claim.

Some objectors complain that the settlement, which may cost the NFL $1 billion over its lifetime, represents a "fraction of one year's revenues." Even so, that does not change the analysis of this *Girsh* factor. Indeed, " 'in any class action against a large corporation, the defendant entity is likely to be able to withstand a more substantial judgment, and, against the weight of the remaining factors, this fact alone does not undermine the reasonableness of the . . . settlement.'" *Sullivan*, 667 F.3d at 323 (quoting *Weber v. Gov't Empl. Ins. Co.*, 262 F.R.D. 431, 447 (D.N.J. 2009)).

7. RANGE OF REASONABLENESS OF THE SETTLEMENT IN LIGHT OF THE BEST POSSIBLE RECOVERY AND ALL ATTENDANT RISKS OF LITIGATION

In evaluating the eighth and ninth *Girsh* factors, we ask "whether the settlement represents a good value for a weak case or a poor value for a strong case."

Warfarin, 391 F.3d at 538. "The factors test two sides of the same coin: reasonableness in light of the best possible recovery and reasonableness in light of the risks the parties would face if the case went to trial." *Id.* "[T]he present value of the damages plaintiffs would likely recover if successful, appropriately discounted for the risk of not prevailing, should be compared with the amount of the proposed settlement." *Prudential*, 148 F.3d at 322 (quotation omitted).

If the retired players were successful in their fraud and negligence claims, they would likely be entitled to substantial damages awards. But we must take seriously the litigation risks inherent in pressing forward with the case. The NFL's pending motion to dismiss and other available affirmative defenses could have left retired players to pursue claims in arbitration or with no recovery at all. Hence we agree with the District Court that the settlement represents a fair deal for the class when compared with a risk-adjusted estimate of the value of plaintiffs' claims. *In re Nat'l Football League Players' Concussion Injury Litig.*, 307 F.R.D. at 395.

Objectors claim that the District Court should have taken into account the costs to class members of the registration and claims administration process because they decrease the "real value" for the class. But these costs are not relevant to the eighth and ninth *Girsh* factors. And in any event the Court assured itself that the claims process was "reasonable in light of the substantial monetary awards . . . and imposes no more requirements than necessary." *Id.* at 396.13 The argument that the settlement's failure to compensate CTE makes it a poor value for the class we discuss separately below.

8. PRUDENTIAL *FACTORS*

The District Court found that the relevant *Prudential* factors also weighed in favor of approving the settlement. *Id.* at 395–96. No objectors engage with the Court's findings on this front. But briefly, we agree that class counsel was able to assess the probable outcome of this case, class members had the opportunity to opt out, and the claims process is reasonable. The provision of attorneys' fees was a neutral factor because class counsel has not yet moved for a fee award.

C. SETTLEMENT'S TREATMENT OF CTE

Objectors raise other arguments about the fairness of the settlement that do not necessarily fall neatly within one of the *Girsh* factors. The most common of those arguments is that the exclusion of CTE as a Qualifying Diagnosis for future claimants is unfair. Objectors note that CTE, the "industrial disease of football," was at the center of the first concussion lawsuits and argue that claims for CTE compensation are released by the settlement in return for nothing. The District Court carefully considered this argument before deciding that the settlement's treatment of CTE was reasonable. It made detailed factual findings about the state of medical science regarding CTE—findings that we review for clear error—in support of this conclusion.

The Court first determined that "[t]he study of CTE is nascent, and the symptoms of the disease, if any, are unknown." *Id.* at 397. Surveying the available medical literature, it found that researchers have not "reliably determined which events make a person more likely to develop CTE" and "have not determined what symptoms individuals with CTE typically suffer from while they are alive." *Id.* at 398. At the time of the Court's decision, only about 200 brains with CTE had been examined, and the only way currently to diagnose CTE is a post-mortem examination of the subject's brain. *Id.*

Citing studies by Dr. Ann McKee and Dr. Robert Stern, objectors argued that CTE progresses in four stages. In Stages I and II, the disease affects mood and behavior while leaving a retired player's cognitive functions largely intact. Headaches, aggression, depression, explosive outbursts, and suicidal thoughts are common. Later in life, as a retired player progresses to Stages III and IV, severe memory loss, dementia, loss of attention and concentration, and impairment of language begin to occur. The District Court explained, however, that these studies suffer from several limitations and cannot generate "[p]redictive, generalizable conclusions" about CTE. *Id.* at 399. The studies suffered from a selection bias because they only examined patients with a history of repetitive head injury. They had to rely on reports by family members to reconstruct the symptoms patients showed before death. And they did not take into account other potential risk factors for developing CTE, including a high Body Mass Index ("BMI"), lifestyle change, age, chronic pain, or substance abuse. *Id.* at 398–99.

With this science in mind, the Court next determined that certain symptoms associated with CTE, such as memory loss, executive dysfunction, and difficulty with concentration, are compensated by the existing Qualifying Diagnoses. *Id.* And many persons diagnosed with CTE after death suffered from conditions in life that are compensated, including ALS, Alzheimer's disease, and Parkinson's disease. Relying on expert evidence, the Court estimated that "at least 89% of the former NFL players" who were examined in CTE studies would have been compensated under the settlement. *Id.*

To be sure, the mood and behavioral symptoms associated with CTE (aggression, depression, and suicidal thoughts) are not compensated, but this result was reasonable. Mood and behavioral symptoms are common in the general population and have multifactor causation and many other risk factors. *Id.* at 401. Retired players tend to have many of these risk factors, such as sleep apnea, a history of drug and alcohol abuse, a high BMI, chronic pain, and major lifestyle changes. *Id.* Class members would thus "face more difficulty proving that NFL Football caused these mood and behavioral symptoms than they would proving that it caused other symptoms associated with Qualifying Diagnoses." *Id.*

The District Court also reviewed the monetary award for post-mortem diagnoses of CTE. It found "[s]ound reasons" for limiting the award to players who died before final approval of the settlement. *Id.* As we have summarized elsewhere, this compensation for deceased players is a proxy for Qualifying Diagnoses a retired player could have received while living. After final approval, players "should be well aware of the [s]ettlement and the need to obtain Qualifying Diagnoses," and "there no longer is a need for Death with CTE to serve as a proxy for Qualifying Diagnoses." *Id.* at 402.

Finally, the Court addressed the potential development of scientific and medical knowledge of CTE. Objectors argued that the settlement's treatment of CTE was unreasonable in light of the expected developments in CTE research. But even if a diagnosis of CTE during life will be available in the next five or ten years, "the longitudinal epidemiological studies necessary to build a robust clinical profile will still take a considerable amount of time." *Id.* The Court also noted that the settlement has some mechanism for keeping pace with science, in that the parties must meet and confer every ten years in good faith about possible modifications to the definitions of Qualifying Diagnoses. *Id.* at 403

Objectors have not shown any of the District Court's findings to be clearly erroneous, which exists when, "although there is evidence to support [the finding], the reviewing court, based on the entire evidence, concludes with firm conviction that a mistake has been made." *GM Trucks*, 55 F.3d at 783. Objectors argue that the Court overlooked certain expert evidence, but the record does not support this contention. They also complain that it failed to weigh the credibility of the different experts when the objectors' experts were not paid for their services. We do not see how the Court could have made a proper credibility determination on the basis of written declarations alone, and, in any event, we have never required those determinations when considering the fairness of a settlement.

Others claim that the expert evidence on CTE should have been analyzed under *Daubert v. Merrell Dow Pharmaceuticals, Inc.*, 509 U.S. 579 (1993), which established threshold standards for the admissibility of expert scientific testimony at trial. Objectors failed to present this argument to the District Court, and we deem it waived. *In re Ins. Brokerage*, 579 F.3d at 261. Moreover, we have never held that district courts, considering the fairness of a class action settlement, should consider the admissibility of expert evidence under *Daubert*. And at least one court of appeals has rejected the argument objectors are making, because "[i]n a fairness hearing, the judge does not resolve the parties' factual disputes but merely ensures that the disputes are real and that the settlement fairly and reasonably resolves the parties' differences." (*Int'l Union, United Auto., Aerospace, & Agr. Implement Workers of Am. v. Gen. Motors Corp.*, 497 F.3d 615, 636–37 [6th Cir. 2007].)

Finding no clear errors in the District Court's findings on CTE, we are also convinced that the Court was well within its discretion in concluding that the settlement's treatment of this condition was reasonable. Most importantly, objectors are not correct when they assert that CTE claims are released by the settlement in return for "nothing." A primary purpose of the settlement is to provide insurance for living players who develop certain neurocognitive or neuromuscular impairments linked to repetitive head trauma (in addition to the benefits provided by the Baseline Assessment Program). Given what we know about CTE, many of the symptoms associated with the disease will be covered by this insurance. And compensation for players who are coping with these symptoms now is surely preferable to waiting until they die to pay their estates for a CTE diagnosis. Moreover, we agree with the District Court that it would be an uphill battle to compensate for the mood and behavioral symptoms thought to be associated with CTE.

Before concluding, we address developments during the pendency of this appeal. In a March 2016 roundtable discussion on concussions organized by the House Energy & Commerce Subcommittee on Oversight & Investigations, the NFL's Executive Vice President cited the research of Dr. McKee and agreed that there was a link between football and degenerative brain disorders like CTE. The NFL's statement is an important development because it is the first time, as far as we can tell, the NFL has publicly acknowledged a connection between football and CTE. On the other hand, the NFL is now conceding something already known. The sheer number of deceased players with a postmortem diagnosis of CTE supports the unavoidable conclusion that there is a relationship, if not a causal connection, between a life in football and CTE.

Objectors cite the NFL's concession as further evidence that this settlement should be rejected. They argue that the NFL has now admitted there is a link between football and CTE, yet refused to compensate the disease. Again, we note that the settlement does compensate many of the impairments associated with CTE, though it does not compensate CTE as a diagnosis (with the exception of players who died before final approval of the settlement). Moreover, even if the NFL has finally come around to the view that there is a link between CTE and football, many more questions must be answered before we could say that the failure to compensate the diagnosis was unreasonable. For example, we still cannot reliably determine the prevalence, symptoms, or risk factors of CTE. The NFL's recent acknowledgment may very well advance the public discussion of the risks of contact sports, but it did not advance the science.

Accordingly, the NFL's statement is not a ground for reversal of the settlement's approval.

In the end, this settlement was the bargain struck by the parties, negotiating amid the fog of litigation. If we were drawing up a settlement ourselves, we may want different terms or more compensation for a certain condition. But our role as judges is to review the settlement reached by the parties for its fairness, adequacy, and reasonableness. And when exercising that role, we must "guard against demanding too large a settlement based on [our] view of the merits of the litigation; after all, settlement is a compromise, a yielding of the highest hopes in exchange for certainty and resolution." (*GM Trucks*, 55 F.3d at 806.) This settlement will provide significant and immediate relief to retired players living with the lasting scars of a NFL career, including those suffering from some of the symptoms associated with CTE. We must hesitate before rejecting that bargain based on an unsupported hope that sending the parties back to the negotiating table would lead to a better deal. Accordingly, we conclude that the settlement's treatment of CTE does not render the agreement fundamentally unfair. We address a few remaining objections to the District Court's fairness inquiry. Some claim that the offsets in the settlement that reduce a player's monetary award were unreasonable. The

Court explained why each offset had scientific support and we are content to say that objectors have not shown its findings to be clearly in error or its conclusions an abuse of discretion. *In re Nat'l Football League Players' Concussion Injury Litig.*, 307 F.R.D. at 407–11. Others argue that the settlement should have used the definition of "eligible season" set forth in the NFL retirement plan. We concur with the District Court that the definition of eligible season in the settlement was reasonable because it is a proxy for the number of head injuries. *Id.* at 410.

VII. Attorneys' Fees

Class counsel and the NFL did not negotiate the issue of fees until after the initial term sheet was signed. After negotiations, the NFL agreed not to contest any award of attorneys' fees and costs up to $112.5 million. Any fee award will be separate from the NFL's obligations under the settlement to pay monetary awards to the retired players. Class counsel may also petition the District Court to set aside 5% of each monetary award to administer the settlement. The petition for a fee award will be submitted to the Court at a later date. Objectors will then be able to present arguments as to why the requested award is improper, and the Court will have discretion to modify the award in whatever way it sees fit. Even though the issue of attorneys' fees remains undecided, some object that the settlement's treatment of fees is a reason for reversal.

A. DEFERRAL OF FEE PETITION

Objectors first argue that the District Court abused its discretion in approving the procedure for attorneys' fees. As noted, class counsel will request a fee award after the class action is certified and the class settlement is approved. Objectors claim that the "attorney-fee-deferral procedure" violated Federal Rule of Civil Procedure Rule 23(h) and deprived class members of due process. We note at the outset that objectors failed to present most of the elements of this argument to the Court at the final fairness hearing. The closest anyone came was when amicus Public Citizen, Inc. claimed that the absence of a fee petition "prevents a complete evaluation of the fairness of the settlement at this point." In response, the Court noted that interested parties would have an opportunity to object to the fee petition when filed and that the separation of settlement approval from fee approval was an "accepted approach." *In re Nat'l Football League Players' Concussion Injury Litig.*, 307 F.R.D. at 396.

As discussed elsewhere, the standards for waiver may be relaxed somewhat in the class action context because we have an independent obligation to protect the rights of absent class members. Applying this principle, we will reach the objections concerning attorneys' fees because, if the objections are persuasive, class members were denied a meaningful chance to object or opt out from the settlement. Our review, however, confirms that the procedure for awarding fees in this settlement was neither an unlawful procedure nor an obstacle to approval. We have no doubt that, at the specified time, class counsel's fee petition will be subject to careful review by the District Court and objectors will present challenges to the fee petition if warranted.

To start, the practice of deferring consideration of a fee award is not so irregular. We have seen the same arrangement in the settlement of a products liability class action related to diet drugs. *In re Diet Drugs Prods. Liab. Litig.*, 582 F.3d 524, 534–35 (3d Cir. 2009) (settlement approved in 2002, interim and final fee awards approved in 2009). Other courts have also used the same procedure. *E.g.*, *In re Oil Spill by Oil Rig Deepwater Horizon in Gulf of Mexico*, 910 F. Supp. 2d 891, 918 (E.D. La. 2012), *aff'd sub nom. In re Deepwater Horizon*, 739 F.3d 790 (5th Cir. 2014); *see also Newberg on Class Actions* § 14:5 (5th ed.) ("In some situations, the court will give final approval to a class action settlement and leave fees and costs for a later determination.").

Moreover, the separation of a fee award from final approval of the settlement does not violate Rule 23(h), which allows a court to award reasonable attorneys' fees and costs in a certified class action subject to certain requirements. Nowhere does the provision require that class counsel move for its fee award at the same time that it moves for final approval of the settlement. Under the Rule, a fee petition must be made by motion served on all parties and, when the motion is made by class counsel, notice must be "directed to class members in a reasonable manner." Fed. R. Civ. P. 23(h)(1). Class members may then object and the court may hold a hearing. Fed. R. Civ. P. 23(h)(2)–(3). And the court "must find the facts and state its legal conclusions" and "may refer issues related to the amount of the award to a special master." Fed. R. Civ. P. 23(h)(3)–(4). So long as these conditions are met, the procedure for awarding attorneys' fees that the District Court approved in this case will not run afoul of subsection (h).

Objectors point us to the Advisory Committee Notes to Rule 23, which seem to contemplate combining class notice of the fee petition with notice of the terms of the settlement. Fed. R. Civ. P. 23(h)(1), 2003 advisory committee's note ("For motions by class counsel in cases subject to court review of a proposed settlement under Rule 23(e), it would be important to require the filing of at least the initial motion in time for inclusion of information about the motion in the notice to the class about the proposed settlement that is required by Rule 23(e).") & ("In cases in which settlement approval is contemplated under Rule 23(e), notice of class counsel's fee motion should be combined with notice of the proposed settlement, and the provision regarding notice to the class is parallel to the requirements for notice under Rule 23(e)."); *see also Newberg on Class Actions* § 8.24 (5th ed.) (Rule 23 envisions "linking together settlement notice and objections with fee notices and objections"). But even if we were willing to read the Advisory Committee's suggestion that fee petitions be filed alongside the settlement as a requirement, "it is the Rule itself, not the Advisory Committee's description of it, that governs." *Dukes*, 131 S. Ct. at 2559.

Objectors also cite as support two cases from other circuits that found a violation of Rule 23(h). *See Redman v. RadioShack Corp.*, 768 F.3d 622, 638 (7th

Cir. 2014), *cert. denied sub nom. Nicaj v. Shoe Carnival, Inc.*, 135 S. Ct. 1429 (2015); *In re Mercury Interactive Corp. Sec. Litig.*, 618 F.3d 988, 993 (9th Cir. 2010). They are not, however, as helpful as objectors might think. In those cases, the district courts denied class members the opportunity to object to the particulars of counsel's fee request because counsel were not required to file a fee petition until after the deadline for class members to object expired. By the time they were served with notice of the fee petition, it was too late for them to object. We have little trouble agreeing that Rule 23(h) is violated in those circumstances. But in our case the fee petition has not yet been filed, the District Court has not set a deadline for objections to the fee petition, and the issue of whether class members will have an opportunity to object is hypothetical. Accordingly, we decline to hold that Rule 23(h) mandates the simultaneous notice of a class action settlement and notice of the fee petition. The final argument raised by objectors on this point is that the decision to delay ruling on the fee award deprived class members of due process. As we discussed in evaluating classwide notice, constitutional due process requires that notice be "reasonably calculated, under all the circumstances, to apprise interested parties of the pendency of the action and afford them an opportunity to present their objections." *Mullane*, 339 U.S. at 314. Put another way, the notice of a class settlement "should contain sufficient information to enable class members to make informed decisions on whether they should take steps." *In re Baby Prods.*, 708 F.3d at 180.

The class notice here was sufficient to comply with due process. The notice advised that the NFL would pay attorneys' fees from a separate fund and not object to an award up to $112.5 million and that the District Court would consider fees after final approval and afford retired players an opportunity to object. From this, class members knew from where the fees for class counsel were coming (a separate fund), what the NFL's position on fees would be (no objection up to $112.5 million), and could ballpark the size of class counsel's eventual fee request (a betting person would say it will be close to $112.5 million). Even if the class members were missing certain information—for example, the number of hours class counsel worked and the terms of any contingency fee arrangements class counsel have with particular retired players—they still had enough information to make an informed decision about whether to object to or opt out from the settlement.

To be sure, we are sympathetic to concerns that others have raised over the practice of delaying consideration of a fee motion. As one treatise put it, [a] primary concern about class action settlements is that unmonitored class counsel may have incentives to sell out the class's interests in return for a large fee. To assess whether such a sell-out has occurred, class members need information *both* about the content of the settlement *and* about the scope of the fee. In this sense, fee notice not only may accompany settlement notice; it likely *should* accompany settlement notice.

Newberg on Class Actions § 8:22 (5th ed.) ([emphases in original].) Delaying the fee petition denies class members information about what their counsel did in negotiating the settlement. And, all else being equal, the more information available the better. Moreover, class members may have less incentive to object to the fee award at a later time because approval of the settlement will have already occurred. But the procedure is not necessarily a violation of Rule 23(h), and in this instance it did not violate due process.

B. CLEAR SAILING PROVISION

Objectors next challenge the provision in the settlement agreement that the NFL would not object to a fee award up to $112.5 million. This is often referred to as a "clear sailing provision" (probably because the implication is that the fee request stands a much better chance of court approval if the defendant is not objecting). The concern with a clear sailing provision is collusion. The defendant is indifferent to the allocation of its liability between the class and counsel; all that matters is the total liability. To forgo the opportunity to object to the fee award, the defendant will presumably want something in return because it is giving up the chance to reduce its overall liability. We thus might fear that class counsel has given away something of value to the class in return for the defendant's agreement not to contest a fee request below a certain level. Despite these concerns, "numerous cases . . . have approved agreements containing such clear-sailing clauses." *In re Oil Spill by Oil Rig Deepwater Horizon*, 295 F.R.D. 112, 138 (E.D. La. 2013). We join our sister circuits in declining to hold that clear sailing provisions are *per se* bars to settlement approval while nonetheless emphasizing that they deserve careful scrutiny in any class action settlement. *See In re Sw. Airlines Voucher Litig.*, 799 F.3d 701, 712 (7th Cir. 2015); *Gooch v. Life Inv'rs Ins. Co. of Am.*, 672 F.3d 402, 426 (6th Cir. 2012); *In re Bluetooth Headset Prods. Liab. Litig.*, 654 F.3d 935, 949 (9th Cir. 2011); *Blessing v. Sirius XM Radio Inc.*, 507 F. App'x 1, 4 (2d Cir. 2012); *Weinberger v. Great N. Nekoosa Corp.*, 925 F.2d 518, 525 (1st Cir. 1991). A district court faced with such a provision in a class action settlement should review the process and substance of the settlement and satisfy itself that the agreement does not indicate collusion or otherwise pose a problem.

The District Court here found the clear sailing provision unobjectionable. It emphasized that the issue of fees was not discussed until after the principal terms of the settlement were agreed to, the fee award will not diminish class recovery, and the agreed amount is just over 10% of the estimated class recovery. *In re Nat'l Football League Players' Concussion Injury Litig.*, 307 F.R.D. at 374–75. We discern no abuse of discretion. There is simply no evidence in the negotiation process or the final terms of the settlement that class counsel bargained away the claims of retired players in return for their own fees.

VIII. Conclusion

It is the nature of a settlement that some will be dissatisfied with the ultimate result. Our case is no different, and we do not doubt that objectors are well-intentioned in making thoughtful arguments against certification of the class and approval of this settlement. They aim to ensure that the claims of retired players are not given up in exchange for anything less than a generous settlement agreement negotiated by very able representatives. But they risk making the perfect the enemy of the good. This settlement will provide nearly $1 billion in value to the class of retired players. It is a testament to the players, researchers, and advocates who have worked to expose the true human costs of a sport so many love. Though not perfect, it is fair.

In sum, we affirm because we are satisfied that the District Court ably exercised its discretion in certifying the class and approving the settlement.

Source: In Re: National Football League Players Concussion Injury Litigation. US Court of Appeals, Third Circuit, Nos. 15–2206, 15–2217, 15–2230, 15–2234, 15–2272, 15–2273, 15–2290, 15–2291, 15–2292, 15–2294, 15–2304 & 15–2305. April 18, 2016.

Timeline

1928   Harrison Martland describes Punch-Drunk Syndrome

1941   Denny-Brown and Russell describe the role of acceleration in the production of concussion

1943   Holburn discusses the respective roles of rotational and linear acceleration in the production of concussion

1973   Corsellis describes the neurological consequences of a career in boxing

1974   Ommaya and Gennarelli resolve continuing dispute about rotational versus linear acceleration in the production of concussion

1975   Gronwall describes the cumulative effects of repeated concussions

1983   Gerberich describes the incidence of sport-related concussion in American football

1984   Saunders and Harbaugh's second impact syndrome initial case report

1986   Cantu recognizes sport-related concussion as potentially more serious than previously thought and develops guidelines for sport-related concussion management

1987   Alves describes the use of neuropsyhological assessments in football

1996   Roberts describes the use of fair play rules for injury reduction in ice hockey

1996   Sosin describes the incidence of concussion in many sports, not just football, for boys and girls

1997   American Academy of Neurology practice parameter for sport-related concussion

1997   McCrea develops sideline assessment; standardized assessment of concussion

1999   Collins paper regarding neuropsyhological assessment of concussion in the *Journal of the American Medical Association*

2001   First international conference on concussion in sport held in Vienna, which describes the role of cognitive and physical rest in recovery and a gradual, stepwise return-to-play after recovery

2003   Guskieiwcz describes the potential cumulative effects of concussions sustained during American football in the *Journal of the American Medical Association*

2004   McCrea describes the underreporting of sport-related concussions by high school football players

2005   Index case of chronic traumatic encephalopathy in a former National Football League player

2007   Centers for Disease Control and Prevention estimate that as many as 1.6–3.8 million nonfatal traumatic brain injuries occur in sports each year in the United States

2007   Former professional wrestler Chris "Harvard" Nowinski publishes his book, *Head Games: Football's Concussion Crisis*, increasing awareness of concussions in sports

2007   Alan Schwartz writes in the *New York Times* about the brain disease of former National Football League player, Andre Waters

2009   Pathologist Ann McKee publishes a large case series of people with chronic traumatic encephalopathy

2010   Leddy describes the introduction of subsymptom threshold exercise to symptomatic patients during recovery from sport-related concussion

2011   Animal models of concussion more analogous to sport-related concussion are introduced to the scientific literature

2014   Collins describes an association between neck strength and risk of sport-related concussion

2015   Kondo A, Mannix R, Lu KP, et al. describe an antibody that blocks abnormal cis tau formation in animals after traumatic brain injuries

2016   The 5th international conference on concussion in sports is scheduled for October in Berlin, Germany

GLOSSARY

While many of the terms used in this book will be well known to its readers, there is some jargon and terms that are unique to sports and athletes, unique to medicine, and some that are unique to sports medicine. In order to ensure correct interpretation and understanding of the text, we will define and describe some of those terms here.

Adenosine Triphosphate: Adenosine triphosphate or ATP consists of an adenosine molecule that is bonded to three phosphate groups. It is the molecule often described as the fuel for the human body. It is the energy molecule of the body. When it undergoes breakdown from ATP to ADP, it releases energy that can be used by the cells of the body to work, helping the heart to pump, the brain to think, the lungs to breathe, and other such functions.

Amnesia: Amnesia is the medical term for the loss of memory. In the setting of sport-related concussion, it refers to a loss of memory due to trauma to the head. Most sport-related concussions do not involve amnesia, and when they do, it is usually of short duration.

Athletic Trainer: An athletic trainer is a medical professional whose expertise is in the assessment, diagnosis, and management of sport-related injuries. At the professional level, all teams will have an athletic trainer that cares for the athletes on that team. This will be true of most college teams as well. When you get down to the high school aged athletes or younger, athletic trainers are less common; about 40 percent of United States high schools have an athletic trainer. Please note that it is an athletic trainer for the school, meaning that many will have only one athletic trainer responsible for multiple teams.

This is significant, as athletic trainers are at the school or team facilities. They are often, when available, the first person to be aware of an injury and to assess it. They often make the diagnosis and the treatment of themselves, but in many states work in collaboration with a sports medicine physician. Athletic trainers are solely focused on sport-related injuries and are often more up to date with the medical literature regarding sports injuries. They can be useful in preparing for catastrophic injuries as well as for preventing injuries by ensuring the teams use proper equipment, and are equipped for proper hydration, nutrition, and maintenance of safe training regimens and protocols.

Catastrophic Injury: A catastrophic injury is a severe injury to the brain or spinal cord that results in death or permanent neurological dysfunction.

Certified Strength and Conditioning Specialist: A certified strength and conditioning specialist is the person who is trained in the techniques used for strengthening the muscles and improving cardiovascular conditioning. They are often employed by teams and athletes to help with training regimens, such that athletes become stronger, faster, more agile, and ultimately more successful in sports.

Clinician: Clinician is a general term for any professional engaged in providing medical care or care to those with illness or injury. Common clinicians treating athletes with sport-related injuries, and sport-related concussion in particular include athletic trainers, nurses, primary care physicians, sports medicine physicians, neurologists, neuropsychologists, psychologists, neurosurgeons, emergency medicine physicians, nurse practitioners, and physician assistants, among others.

Cognition/Cognitive Function: The term cognition is a medical word used to describe functions of the brain that involve thinking, reasoning, concentrating, and learning. Cognition is a blanket term used to describe those aspects of brain function. Most of the things we do consciously with our brains involve cognition. Common tasks that involve cognition include reading, schoolwork or homework, playing board games or video games, doing crossword puzzles, and other similar activities.

Collision Sports: Collision sports are those in which intentional body to body blows and tackling are an allowed part of the game and indeed part of the rules. Common collision sports include American football, rugby, men's ice hockey, men's lacrosse, and Australian rules football, among others.

Combat Sports: Combat sports are a subclassification of collision sports that involve an actual fighting, albeit a controlled fight within a specific set of rules and regulations. Common combat sports include boxing, wrestling, mixed martial arts, karate, and other similar activities.

Computerized Neurocognitive Assessment: Computerized neurocognitive assessments are measures of brain function performed on a computer. In the setting of sport-related concussion, they are often used to obtain baseline measures of brain function. Those baseline measures are often compared to measures taken postinjury to assess any degree of change in cognitive function of athletes after concussion. They also used to monitor recovery of cognitive function among athletes to determine when they have returned to their prior preinjury baseline.

Contact Sports: Contact sports are those sports in which incidental contact with another player is an expected and anticipated part of the game; however, intentional body to body blows and tackling are not allowed. Some common contact sports include soccer, basketball, and baseball, among others.

Diagnosis: Diagnosis refers to the act of identifying a disease, illness, or injury by examining a patient. When athletes see the doctor after sustaining a blow to the head that is associated with nausea, dizziness, headaches, and difficulty concentrating, they are diagnosed with a concussion.

Epidemiology: Epidemiology is the study of the distribution and determinants of disease, injury, or illness. Epidemiology is the study of the frequency of disease as well as the causes of increased or decreased frequency of disease, injury, or illness.

Hyperphosphorylated Tau/Cis Tau: Tau is a normal protein found in the brain that is used for the stabilization of an organelle known as a microtubule. Hyperphosphorylated tau and cis tau are abnormal forms of tau that are associated with repeated trauma to the brain. Hyperphosphorylated tau is used for the definition of chronic traumatic encephalopathy, which is currently defined as the presence of hyperphosphorylated tau in a specific distribution.

Imaging: In medicine, imaging is a way of obtaining pictures of various parts of the body. Most readers will know that an X-ray allows the doctor to visualize the bones of the body. It is a very common form of imaging used in medicine. But X-rays are not as useful for the imaging of potential brain injuries. Although concussion cannot currently be seen on most forms of modern-day imaging, computed tomography (CT) and magnetic resonance images (MRIs) are often used to ensure there are no additional or other injuries that might explain athletes symptoms, essentially ruling out other injuries in order to make the diagnosis of concussion.

Incidence: In epidemiology, the study of injury, illness, or disease, the term incidence refers to the occurrence of an injury, illness, or disease over a given time period, most often a year. For example, if there are one million sport-related concussions each year in the United States, it could be said that "the incidence of sport-related concussion in the United States is one million per year."

Neurobehavioral: The term neurobehavioral refers to the interaction between the nerves of the body and behavior. In the setting of sport-related concussion, it refers to the way concussion affects the nerves, thereby affecting behavior, or perhaps the way cumulative effects of multiple concussions can cause changes to the nerves and behavior later in life, including chronic traumatic encephalopathy.

Neuromuscular: The term neuromuscular refers to the interaction between the nerves and the muscles, of the way the nerves control the normal action and movement of the muscles.

Neuropsychologist: A neuropsychologist is a clinician and scientist whose specialty is in the realm of brain function. Neuropsychologists are doctors of philosophy or doctors of psychology who have gone on to train and care for patients with disorders of brain function. Neuropsychologists are used in performing baseline as well as postinjury neuropsychological assessment on athletes who are suspected of having sustained sport-related concussions. Neuropsychologists are the professionals who developed computerized neurocognitive measures, also referred to in this book.

Often, athletes who sustain sport-related concussions and are either slow to recover or have profound cognitive difficulties will be sent to a neuropsychologist for evaluation. During that evaluation, the neuropsychologist is able to better characterize the degree of cognitive dysfunction of the athlete, if any, and elucidate possible contributing factors and causes of that dysfunction.

Neurologist: A neurologist is a doctor who specializes in treating disorders, diseases, and illnesses that affect the nerves of the body and brain. Classically, sport-related concussion was not a part of neurology training and was not an injury seen by most neurologists. There has been, however, a concerted effort over the last several years to train neurologists in the assessment and management of this injury and calls for them to play a bigger role in the area. This should be welcomed, given the number of concussions that occur each year. Nowadays, many if not most neurologists will be familiar with the assessment and management recommendations for concussion. Those who are not will likely have a colleague that they can refer patients to for such care.

Neurosurgeon: A neurosurgeon is a surgeon whose expertise is in surgeries of the brain, spinal cord, central nervous system, and surrounding structures. Although sport-related concussion is not an indication for surgery, neurosurgeons are often the ones who respond to trauma and, therefore, often play a role in the assessment and management of sport-related concussion.

Noncontact Sports: Noncontact sports are those in which the participating athletes do not make contact with each other as an anticipated or expected part of the game. Common noncontact sports are cross-country running, track and field, tennis, golf, and swimming, among others.

Nurse Practitioner: A nurse practitioner is a registered nurse who has gone on to do extra medical training. Nurse practitioners are able to evaluate patients, order medical studies, make diagnoses, and prescribe treatments, including prescription medications. In many states, nurse practitioners operate under the license of a supervising physician; however, they often function independently. They act in many ways similar to a physician but have not undergone the same degree of training and do not have a medical doctorate.

Ocular: Ocular is a medical adjective used to describe things associated with the eyes or with vision.

Pathophysiology: Pathophysiology is the science of abnormal physiology. That is to say, pathophysiology describes the abnormal processes of organs and organisms when they are injured, diseased, or ill.

Personal Trainer: Personal trainer is a less specific term used to define someone who contributes to the overall training regimen and physical conditioning of an athlete. Many personal trainers are certified strength and conditioning specialists but not all of them.

Physician Assistant: Like a nurse practitioner, a physician assistant has undergone training that allows him or her to assess patients, order medical studies, make diagnoses, and administer treatments for those diagnoses. A physician assistant acts in many ways like a physician, but has not undergone the same degree of training that a medical doctor has and does not have a medical doctorate.

Physiology: Physiology is the science that involves the normal functions of living organisms and organs. Physiology is a branch of biology that describes the normal functioning of organisms and organs. The way the brain normally functions and conducts signals would be normal brain physiology.

Primary Care Physician: A primary care physician is most closely associated with the patient. It is the doctor from whom patients receive their regular physical examinations. It is the doctor who coordinates all aspects of the patient care and often coordinates specialty care when it is indicated. Primary care physicians are trained in the primary care specialties such as internal medicine, family practice, or pediatrics. They are very important in the diagnosis and management of sport-related concussion and often are the main doctor caring for athletes who sustain sport-related concussions.

Prognosis: The term prognosis refers to a prediction or judgment, most often by a doctor, about the future of an injury, illness, or disease. In setting sport-related concussion, the prognosis involves predicting the time it will take the athlete to recover.

Psychiatrist: A psychiatrist is a medical doctor who specializes in the assessment and management of mental illness. They can often be used in conjunction with a psychologist or independently to treat some of the underlying conditions that occur with concussion or as a result of the treatment of concussion. They can prescribe medications when needed.

Psychologist: A clinician who specializes in treating emotional and behavioral disorders without medication but with other forms of therapy is known as a psychologist. Some psychologists have specialized in the psychological problems faced by athletes and are known as sports psychologists. In the realm of sport-related concussion, sports psychologists are often useful in helping athletes cope with longer recoveries, recognize other contributing factors to their overall symptoms, reassuring them regarding recovery, and administering treatment for associated depression, anxiety, or other psychological problems.

Risk Factor: A risk factor is a factor or variable that is associated with an increased risk of disease, injury, or illness. For example, cigarette smoking is a strong risk factor for lung cancer.

Second Impact Syndrome: Second impact syndrome describes the phenomenon whereby an athlete who is not yet fully recovered from a sport-related concussion sustains an additional blow to the head, often a mild one, which is associated with massive swelling of the brain and often death. It is a rare occurrence.

Signs: Medical professionals often refer to the signs of an injury, illness, or disease. Signs of an illness, injury, or disease are those characteristics that can be observed by the doctor or by other people who are observing the patient. Gross imbalance, repetitive questioning, loss of consciousness are some signs of concussion that can be observed when an athlete has sustained a sport-related concussion.

Sports Medicine Doctor: A sports medicine doctor is a doctor who has completed training and is certified in the field of sports medicine. There are two main branches of sports medicine. The first one derived from family practice, but has expanded since to other medical specialties. Physicians certified under this pathway will have trained initially in internal medicine, family practice, pediatrics, emergency medicine, or physical medicine and rehabilitation. They will have gone on to do a fellowship in sports medicine and have passed the test certifying them as a sports medicine physician.

Alternatively, orthopedic surgeons may undergo a subspecialization in sports medicine. Orthopedic surgeons who have done this will have trained and performed surgeries for injuries that are common among athletes, in ways that allow athletes return-to-play sooner after their surgery, particularly arthroscopy, which involves putting a cannula, or arthroscope, into a joint in order to perform surgery as opposed to opening up the joint entirely.

Symptom Inventory: Often, the symptoms of concussion are measured and quantified using what is known as a symptom inventory. A symptom inventory consists of a list of the common symptoms of concussion followed by a rating scale on which athletes rate the severity of each symptom. Common symptom inventories include the Rivermead post-concussion symptom questionnaire, the post-concussion symptom scale, and the post-concussion symptom inventory, among others.

Symptoms: Symptoms represent the characteristics of injury, illness, or disease as experienced by the patients themselves. They are not necessarily observable by others but are known to the patient. Common symptoms caused by concussion are headaches, nausea, dizziness, and difficulty with concentration, among others.

Variable: In the study of injury, illness, or disease, also known as epidemiology, the term "variable" refers to a factor that may change between or among people that somehow is related to health.

Vestibular: The vestibular system refers to a system of the body that involves the brain, the eyes, the inner ear, and is ultimately responsible, in part, for controlling balance, coordination, and eye movements. Sport-related concussion can result in disruption of the vestibular system.

Sources for Further Information

Books

Bailes JE, Lovell MR, Maroon JC. *Sports-Related Concussion.* St. Louis, MO: Quality Medical Publishing, Inc., 1999.

Cantu RC, Hyman M. *Concussions and Our Kids: America's Leading Expert on How to Protect Young Athletes and Keep Sports Safe.* Boston, MA: Houghton Mifflin Harcourt, 2012.

Echemendia RJ. *Sports Neuropsychology: Assessment and Management of Traumatic Brain Injury.* New York: The Guilford Press, 2006.

Lovell MR, Echemendia RJ, Barth JT, Collins MW. *Traumatic Brain Injury in Sports.* Lisse, The Netherlands: Swets and Zeitlinger, 2004.

McCrea M. *Mild Traumatic Brain Injury and Postconcussion Syndrome: The New Evidence Base for Diagnosis and Treatment.* New York: Oxford University Press, 2008.

Meehan WP III. *Kids, Sports, and Concussion: A Guide for Coaches and Parents.* Santa Barbara, Denver, and Oxford: Praeger Publishers, 2011

Nowinski C. *Head Games: Football's Concussion Crisis.* East Bridgewater, MA: The Drummond Publishing Group, 2007.

Websites

Brain Injury Association of America—Concussion Information Center (http://www.biausa.org/concussion/concussion-information-center).

Heads Up—Centers for Disease Control and Prevention training on concussion (http://www.cdc.gov/HeadsUp/).

Mom's Team Youth Sports Concussion Safety Center (http://www.momsteam.com/).

ARTICLES

Alves WM, Rimel RW, Nelson WE. University of Virginia prospective study of football-induced minor head injury: status report. *Clin Sports Med.* Jan 1987; 6(1): 211–218.

Aubry M, Cantu R, Dvorak J, et al. Summary and agreement statement of the First International Conference on Concussion in Sport, Vienna 2001. Recommendations for the Corsellis JA, Bruton CJ, Freeman-Browne D. The aftermath of boxing. *Psychol Med.* Aug 1973; 3(3): 270–303.

Brown NJ, Mannix RC, O'Brien MJ, Gostine D, Collins MW, Meehan WP, III. Effect of cognitive Activity level on duration of post-concussion symptoms. *Pediatrics* 2014 Feb; 133(2): e299–304. Collins MW, Grindel SH, Lovell MR, et al. Relationship between concussion and neuropsychological performance in college football players. *JAMA.* Sep 8, 1999; 282(10): 964–970.

Denny-Brown D, Russell R. Experimental cerebral concussion. *Brain.* 1941; 64: 93–164.

Eisenberg MA, Andrea J, Meehan W, Mannix R. Time interval between concussions and symptom duration. *Pediatrics.* Jul 2013; 132(1): 8–17.

Field M, Collins MW, Lovell MR, Maroon J. Does age play a role in recovery from sports-related concussion? A comparison of high school and collegiate athletes. *J Pediatr.* May 2003; 142(5): 546–553.

Gerberich SG, Priest JD, Boen JR, Straub CP, Maxwell RE. Concussion incidences and severity in secondary school varsity football players. *Am J Public Health.* Dec 1983; 73(12): 1370–1375.

Giza CC, Hovda DA. The Neurometabolic Cascade of Concussion. *J Athl Train.* Sep 2001; 36(3): 228–235.

Gronwall D, Wrightson P. Cumulative effect of concussion. *Lancet.* Nov 22, 1975; 2(7943): 995–997.

Guskiewicz KM, McCrea M, Marshall SW, et al. Cumulative effects associated with recurrent concussion in collegiate football players: the NCAA Concussion Study. *JAMA.* Nov 19, 2003; 290(19): 2549–2555.

Guskiewicz KM, Perrin DH, Gansneder BM. Effect of mild head injury on postural stability in athletes. *J Athl Train.* Oct 1996; 31(4): 300–306.

Holbourn A. Mechanics of head Injury. *Lancet.* Oct 9, 1943; 2: 438–441.

Jordan BD, Relkin NR, Ravdin LD, Jacobs AR, Bennett A, Gandy S. Apolipoprotein E epsilon4 associated with chronic traumatic brain injury in boxing. *JAMA.* Jul 9, 1997; 278(2): 136–140.

Leddy JJ, Kozlowski K, Donnelly JP, Pendergast DR, Epstein LH, Willer B. A preliminary study of subsymptom threshold exercise training for refractory post-concussion syndrome. *Clin J Sport Med.* Jan 2010; 20(1): 21–27.

Martland H. Punch drunk. *JAMA.* 1928; 91(15): 1103–1107.

Matser EJ, Kessels AG, Lezak MD, Jordan BD, Troost J. Neuropsychological impairment in amateur soccer players. *JAMA.* Sep 8, 1999; 282(10): 971–973.

McCrea M, Kelly JP, Kluge J, Ackley B, Randolph C. Standardized assessment of concussion in football players. *Neurology.* Mar 1997; 48(3): 586–588.

McCrory P. Does second impact syndrome exist? *Clin J Sport Med.* Jul 2001; 11(3): 144–149.

McCrory P, Meeuwisse W, Aubry M, et al. Consensus statement on concussion in sport—the 4th International Conference on Concussion in Sport held in Zurich, November 2012. *Clin J Sport Med.* Mar 2013; 23(2): 89–117.

McCrory PR, Berkovic SF. Second impact syndrome. *Neurology.* Mar 1998; 50(3): 677–683.

McCrory P, Meeuwisse W, Johnston K, et al. Consensus statement on concussion in sport: the 3rd International Conference on Concussion in Sport held in Zurich, November 2008. *Br J Sports Med.* May 2009; 43 Suppl 1: i76–90.

McKee AC, Cantu RC, Nowinski CJ, et al. Chronic traumatic encephalopathy in athletes: progressive tauopathy after repetitive head injury. *J Neuropathol Exp Neurol.* Jul 2009; 68(7): 709–735.

Meehan WP, III, Mannix RC, O'Brien M J, Collins MW. The prevalence of undiagnosed concussions in athletes. *Clin J Sport Med.* May 30, 2013; Epub ahead of print.

Meehan WP, III, Mannix RC, Stracciolini A, Elbin RJ, Collins MW. Symptom severity predicts prolonged recovery after sport-related concussion, but age and amnesia do not. *J Pediatr.* Sep 2013; 163(3): 721–725.

Meehan WP, III, Mannix R, Monuteaux MC, Stein CJ, Bachur RG. Early symptom burden predicts recovery after sport-related concussion. *Neurology.* 2014 Dec 9; 83(24): 2204–2210.

Meehan WP, III, d'Hemecourt P, Collins CL, Taylor AM, Comstock RD. Computerized neurocognitive testing for the management of sport-related concussions. *Pediatrics.* Jan 2012; 129(1): 38–44.

Meehan WP, III, Zhang J, Khuman J, Mannix R, Whalen MJ. A murine model of multiple mild concussive brain injuries and the effects of recovery time on cognitive outcome. Platform presentation at the National Neurotrauma Symposium, Fort Lauderdale, FL, 2011.

Meehan WP, III, Zhang J, Mannix R, Whalen MJ. Increasing recovery time between injuries improves cognitive outcome after repetitive mild concussive brain injuries in mice. *Neurosurgery.* Oct 2012; 71(4): 885–891.

Moser RS, Glatts C, Schatz P. Efficacy of immediate and delayed cognitive and physical rest for treatment of sports-related concussion. *J Pediatr.* Nov 2012; 161(5): 922–926.

Omalu BI, DeKosky ST, Minster RL, Kamboh MI, Hamilton RL, Wecht CH. Chronic traumatic encephalopathy in a National Football League player. *Neurosurgery.* Jul 2005; 57(1): 128–134; discussion 128–134.

Ommaya AK, Gennarelli TA. Cerebral concussion and traumatic unconsciousness. Correlation of experimental and clinical observations of blunt head injuries. *Brain.* Dec 1974; 97(4): 633–654.

Saunders RL, Harbaugh RE. The second impact in catastrophic contact-sports head trauma. *JAMA.* Jul 27, 1984; 252(4): 538–539.

Shaw NA. The neurophysiology of concussion. *Prog Neurobiol.* Jul 2002; 67(4): 281–344.

Sosin DM, Sniezek JE, Thurman DJ. Incidence of mild and moderate brain injury in the United States, 1991. *Brain Inj.* Jan 1996; 10(1): 47–54.

Talavage TM, Nauman EA, Breedlove EL, et al. Functionally-detected cognitive impairment in high school football players without clinically-diagnosed concussion. *J Neurotrauma.* Feb 15, 2014; 31(4): 327–338.

Van Kampen DA, Lovell MR, Pardini JE, Collins MW, Fu FH. The "value added" of neurocognitive testing after sports-related concussion. *Am J Sports Med.* Oct 2006; 34(10): 1630–1635.

REFERENCES

Beauchamp TL, Childress JF. *Nonmaleficence. Principles of Biomedical Ethics.* New York: Oxford University Press, 1994.

Emery C, Kang J, Shrier I, et al. Risk of injury associated with bodychecking experience among youth hockey players. *CMAJ.* Aug 9, 2011; 183(11):1249–1256.

Guskiewicz KM, Marshall SW, et al. Association between recurrent concussion and late-life cognitive impairment in retired professional football players. *Neurosurgery.* Oct 2005; 57(4):719–726; discussion 719–726.

Zillmer EA, Shneider J, Tinker J, Kaminaris CI. "Chapter 2. A history of sports-related concussions" in Echemendia RJ. *Sports Neuropsychology: Assessment and Management of Traumatic Brain Injury.* New York: The Guilford Press, 2006.

INDEX

About the Author

William Paul Meehan III, MD, is director of the Micheli Center for Sports Injury Prevention, co-director of the Football Players Health Study at Harvard University, and director of research for the Brain Injury Center at Boston Children's Hospital. He graduated from Harvard Medical School, where he is currently an assistant professor of pediatrics and orthopedics. Dr. Meehan is board certified in sports medicine. He conducts both clinical and scientific research in the area of sports injuries, sports injury prevention, and concussive brain injury. His research has been funded by the National Institutes of Health, the National Football League, the National Hockey League Alumni Association, and the Center for the Integration of Medicine and Innovative Technology. He is the 2012 winner of the American Medical Society for Sports Medicine's award for Best Overall Research. He has multiple medical and scientific publications and served as guest editor for the January 2011 issue of *Clinics in Sports Medicine* regarding concussion in sports. He is author of Praeger's *Kids, Sports, and Concussion: A Guide for Coaches and Parents*.